Michael Chapman

Rethinking dementia: ripples and responses

. . . . . .

To the traditional owners of the lands on which
I write and work, the Ngunnawal and Ngambri people,
thank you for your ongoing custody of this amazing country
and for all that you've done and do to enable and support
our community.

Michael Chapman

Rethinking dementia:
ripples and responses

Illustrations: Mirranda Burton

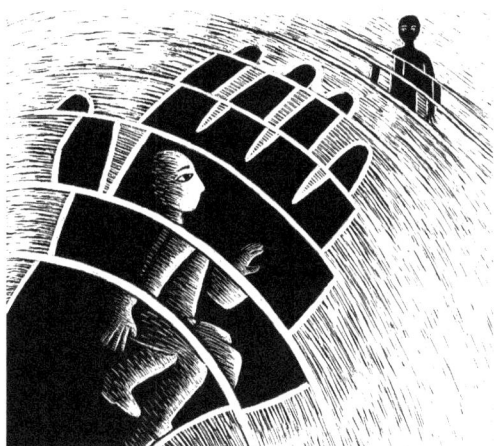

PALAVER

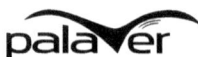

palaver

www.palaver.com
Palaver is an imprint of Ethica Projects Pty. Ltd.
10 Barnato Grove Armadale Victoria 3143 Australia

Contents

Foreword Steven R. Sabat

For most of the 118 years since Alois Alzheimer discovered what he called "a peculiar disease of the cerebral cortex", closely followed in the succeeding years by Emil Kraepelin naming the disease after Alzheimer, the Alzheimer's type of the syndrome called dementia has been understood and treated principally from a medical perspective: as a disease of the person diagnosed. Alzheimer's disease (AD) accounts for the majority of people diagnosed with dementia and leads to serious difficulties in the lives of people diagnosed as well as those of their families, friends, and communities.

As a disease, it has been understood primarily in biomedical terms defined by its symptoms and associated effects on neurophysiological, neurochemical, and neuroanatomical systems. And, given the biomedical approach, the long-established way to treat a disease is to find a preventive measure or a cure because this approach has worked admirably in connection with many other diseases (e.g., polio, malaria). Unfortunately, the search for a cure for AD continues unrequited and the most recent approaches to slowing its progress have been controversial in terms of their safety, efficacy, and cost. To make matters still more complicated, even if there were a biomedical intervention that could stop AD in its tracks and prevent further damage, there would still be millions of people worldwide already diagnosed who would continue to live with the effects of the brain damage that AD caused and still other millions who would develop it because there is no vaccine that would prevent its occurrence.

As if the situation weren't dire already, AD is only one of many diseases (e.g., Parkinson's, HIV, Vascular diseases) that can cause brain damage leading to the syndrome (a group of symptoms) that has been termed *dementia*. "Curing dementia", therefore, requires a cure for each of the diseases that cause the brain damage leading to the syndrome. With this as background, readers will appreciate the reasons behind the thinking and approach offered by Dr. Michael Chapman in this book.

Specifically, he proposes a "systems approach" to understanding and dealing with the rippling effects of dementia because the effects of a person's brain damage are not limited to that particular person, for that person's family and friends are also affected greatly. As well, the person's primary care physician (GP) and consultants/specialists (neurologists, psychiatrists) and other healthcare professionals (e.g., neuropsychologists, nurses, clinical social workers), and communities (e.g., respite centres, dementia cafés, houses of worship) are also affected as they are involved in the assessment, care, and support of people diagnosed and their families. These are only parts of what Dr. Chapman refers to as the many "rippling effects" of dementia that extend well beyond the person diagnosed. Indeed, local, state, and federal governments and private charities are also affected as they are involved in the appropriation of funds and creation of venues to serve the needs of all concerned. And, at a still larger circle of "ripples" are the people whose taxes are collected and then used toward realising many of these efforts.

As there are many "systems" involved with dementia, a *coordinated* "systems approach" is necessary to achieve optimum care and treatment. A first step in creating an encompassing, system-wide culture of care is that the "otherness" of the person diagnosed must cease to be his or her principal defining attribute as it has been all too often. Rather, sharp focus must be maintained also on the many valued human qualities he or she continues to share with others deemed healthy. Thus, there can be no "us" and no "them", but only "we", because "we" are all involved. Dr. Chapman illustrates this point with vivid examples of people diagnosed, their family carers and health care professionals, and the related important and often rather complex psychological and social dynamics that make the experience of people diagnosed and that of others involved challenging to say the least.

Changing the culture of care requires something reminiscent of the operation of two processes that psychologist Jean Piaget observed in the cognitive development of children: *assimilation* and *accommodation*. The former is the process by which we add new information and experience to our existing structures of knowledge, or schemata. Thus, for example, the traditional biomedical schema to deal with disease is to find cures or vaccines and to treat people symptomatically in circumscribed, professional ways. As this approach has worked well in the past, it is applied now to AD and other types of dementia. Accommodation, on the other hand, is the process of changing one's current way of thinking so as to adapt to a new environment. The "new" environment requires recognising that "treatment" must go well beyond the traditional biomedical approach/ schema.

Thus, Dr. Chapman essentially asks, "What form might this new environment for treatment take?" For one thing, it requires sustained education through many systems of communication for carers of all kinds (professionals, families) regarding the cognitive and social strengths still possessed by those diagnosed and ways to use those strengths to everyone's advantage through sensitive communication in words and actions. For example, people living with Alzheimer's disease do not have "memory loss" because they can still make new memories and learn new things. How they express that learning is not by *recalling* this or that event, but by *acting as if they had* learned this or that, especially in response to others' positive or negative treatment that they cannot specifically recall in detail. This is evidenced by the ability of people living with the Alzheimer's type of dementia to enjoy new positive relationships and make new friends.

Furthermore, systems can and should evolve so that professional and family carers engage in mutually supportive relationships that go beyond the currently circumscribed biomedical level. Such relationships must involve carers becoming increasingly understanding of and compassionate about the experience and point of view of people living with dementia, including their feelings of vulnerability, anxiety, sadness, and frustration. People at all levels of social life, including mass media and government representatives, need to be educated about the quintessential importance of creating positive, respectful relationships with people living with dementia. Such relationships go well beyond "daily care" or "managing patients", for they are life enhancing: they make for good moments, the positive rippling effects of which can be seen in physiological, psychological, and social systems.

Thus, Dr. Chapman advocates for a crucial change in the way we understand and interact with our families, friends, neighbours, clients, and patients who are living with one or another form of dementia so that our collective lives may be improved via the recognition and engagement of our collective, common humanity.

Steven R. Sabat PhD
Professor Emeritus of Psychology
Georgetown University
Washington DC 20057 U.S.A.

Rethinking dementia

Introduction

This book is about dementia. In itself, that may not seem particularly noteworthy. There are many excellent books explaining dementia from the perspective of medical science. There are books about the experience of dementia from the vantage of those providing care as clinicians or family and friends of the person with the diagnosis. There are also books explaining the experience written by or alongside people with dementia. While having some things in common with those books, being "about" dementia, for example, this book is a little different. To give some sense of how, I'll share a story about someone whom I will call "Nellie".

Nellie was a mum. Of course, there was a lot more to Nellie. There had been many shared and quiet parts to Nellie over her life. But Nellie thought of herself as a mum. The early chapters of Nellie's time as a mum had been even more exciting and challenging than is true for most parents. She'd travelled with her young family to Papua New Guinea for her husband's work. Talking about this over fifty years later in Melbourne, her kids, Mike and Joan, still bubbled with their delight and wonder at the experience. Back then, and even with all the excitement, Nellie had been able to hold them balanced, letting her kids experience the opportunities of a city and country that were completely new, while also remaining a reminder of the safe and the familiar.

By the time I met Nellie and her family she was in her eighties, and she had dementia. In retrospect, Nellie had managed to mask her symptoms for a number of years before her dementia was diagnosed. Mike and Joan had noticed that Nellie seemed a "little off" over time. Making the meals that Nellie always prided herself on slowly became a drama or a strange impossibility. Nellie often seemed confused and got lost when she was driving in familiar places. She'd also become uncharacteristically forgetful and seemed to struggle to keep track of bookings and events. Eventually this even included things that were a central habit like remembering to get ready for Church. Her family and friends supported her as much as they could and then organised extra carers to support her when that wasn't enough. It was years into this process before they had a term, dementia, to describe what was happening to Nellie. By that time, everyone involved in trying to keep Nellie safe and living independently was exhausted. Worried for her, for themselves, and now feeling that life alone would only become less safe for Nellie, Joan and Mike had begun the process that would ultimately result in Nellie living in a care facility.

When I met her, Nellie was living in a high care facility. I was immediately struck by how warm and companionable Nellie was. She was quick to laugh and liked spending time with other people. Nellie needed a lot of routine help with normal activities like getting dressed or going to the toilet, but she was able to walk by herself and really enjoyed doing this. Her main activity was exploring and re-exploring her environment. She'd wander around the spaces within the facility talking about what she saw with whoever she was with. It was a challenge knowing exactly what Nellie was trying to communicate. Her speech was unclear and fragmented, her words seeming to skip around meaning. But it was clear that Nellie was communicating something. She would repeatedly express what it was she was experiencing and what it meant to her using the language that she had. These moments were clearly important and meaningful for Nellie, but they also seemed incredibly fragile, quickly lost if there was no one with her trying to recognise and make sense of what she was trying to say.

Mike and Joan felt guilty. Partly for "being conned" by Nellie and missing the signs of her dementia that she'd managed to cover over for so long, and for not being able to support her to continue to be the "Nellie" that they and many others remembered. They also felt that by needing to "chuck her" into care they'd failed her in a deep way made worse by knowing how much she'd worked at and treasured being a mother for them well into their adulthood. Seeing Nellie change and "crumbling like plastic in the sun" was tragic for them, a continuing, aching loss. They felt that the "shutters were down" for her now and they desperately wanted to do all that they could to hold on to and treasure all that she had been and what she had valued. They also worried that Nellie was suffering. They knew that she wasn't "the full quid" anymore but they worried that she knew that they lied to her to make it easier for them to leave and go home after their visits. Mike and Joan felt powerless to help Nellie themselves, and so they were determined to make sure that the staff at the facility were doing a good job in caring for their mum.

This had led to them losing their tempers with staff members and criticising the care that they were providing. Talking with them, I could feel how angry they'd been and how distressed they'd felt at how they'd expressed these feelings at the facility. Mike and Joan thought of themselves as good Christians, and they struggled with the compromising necessity of needing to "fight" to ensure that their mum was being cared for in the way she deserved.

Kylie, a senior manager and the care manager at the facility, was another central person in Nellie's, Mike's and Joan's story. Kylie was in charge of the staff who cared for Nellie. Kylie was deeply aware of how challenging these moments were for everyone. Being able to turn up and be helpful required warmth and generosity, qualities which you could feel that Kylie thoughtfully prepared in herself each day, like a neat little lunchbox, knowing that they would be needed. She felt called to working with people with dementia and felt she understood some of what they experienced. When residents like Nellie wandered, she understood that it was because they had somewhere they wanted to be, and when they were agitated, she could see that it was because they were trying to communicate their distress or discomfort to those around them. For Kylie, caring meant always working to understand what this faltering communication meant and being able to respond appropriately. Kylie considered the facility to be Nellie's home and that as a home it needed to be nurturing for Nellie, for her family and for the staff providing care. Kylie respected and admired Mike's and Joan's attempts to maintain normality for Nellie but wondered whether their attempts to do this were more important for them than for her. She also felt that their frustration and grief were increased by their attempts to control her care at the facility and the inexorable changes occurring for Nellie. Kylie believed that the family's actions probably contributed to Nellie's initial agitation and distress at the facility. However, she remained optimistic that the relationship between Mike, Joan and the staff was improving, and that the facility could be a home for Nellie.

What I am calling "Nellie's story" above, and other "stories" to follow, are based on interviews I conducted as part of my research undertaken with people with dementia, their family members and carers, and the clinicians involved in their care. These stories illustrate why we need to think about dementia in new ways.

Dementia is a syndrome, a cluster of problems arising from a variety of potential causes that an individual is diagnosed with. However, its effects are broader. Dementia does not just affect a person, it affects people. The impact of dementia ripples outwards like a stone dropped into a deep, still pond. Nellie has dementia and her condition has advanced to the point where she requires full-time care and lives a very different life now than previously. However, the people expressing the most grief and distress are her children. Far from being a condition of a single individual, dementia impacts families, groups and communities.

Part of my inspiration for writing this book is my awareness that dementia has certainly affected *me*. Early in my medical career, my experience with the challenges of dementia care and my wish to understand dementia and to care for those people with dementia with more skill and compassion affected me deeply. I spent years working in hospitals, in the community and in aged care facilities. I saw people living with and dying from dementia in so many contexts and saw the deep and pervasive tragedy of dementia on so many people. But I also saw that dementia can still include joy, it can still include wonder, it can still include learning and growth. It was largely my experience of caring for people with dementia that led me to train as a geriatrician and as a palliative medicine specialist and to undertake research into aged and dementia care. I humbly hope that my work might make a small contribution to our shared experience of dementia, might diminish some of the dark moments and help make the bright ones clearer and more sustained.

Another somewhat surprising implication from Nellie's story is that not only does dementia affect groups of people, but people touched by dementia directly and indirectly affect how dementia is experienced. People respond to the ripples of dementia. Despite Nellie's changing needs, a community of people supported her to be at home, lessening or covering up dementia's deeper impacts for her for as long as they could. In the care facility, Nellie's exploration, her trying to make sense of and express her experience of her world, was highly dependent on others. Thinking about those fragile, "crumbling" moments, holding them with hope and wonder, sustains the possibility of their value. We're doing that together right now, allowing Nellie to have an impact on us and others. Kylie noted that Mike's and Joan's feelings of guilt for the changes in their mum accounts for their unsustainable expectations of the care staff and contributes to increasing Nellie's agitation and distress. Dementia, it seems, involves a process of interconnected changes within groups of people affected by the diagnosis. This is on one hand a fairly simple and straightforward idea. Dementia is clearly something with a big impact and it doesn't seem a stretch to think that there might be more to it than we usually assume. On the other hand, understanding dementia as an experience involving networks or communities of people actually has huge implications. Thinking about dementia in this way will require us to rethink what we mean when we say "dementia", what "having dementia" means for a person and for those around them and how to respond to it. In this book, we will begin the task of thinking all this through, and what it might mean to do so.

There are a number of good reasons for us to be rethinking dementia now. Dementia's challenge to our society is a big one and it continues to grow. It confronts and challenges so much of how we value and make sense of our ageing and our experience. Key things that we consider important about ourselves like our personhood and our autonomy seem rocked by dementia in ways that many people feel result in a hopeless decline. It's also clear that the tools that drive our current responses to dementia are not working. The usual tools we use to do something when dementia arrives include things like medications, education, care and support approaches, and clinical and legal tools to allow ongoing decision-making if a person no longer has the capacity to do this themselves. These tools are insufficient, but I'd also argue that considering dementia as an experience of communities means that they are also too narrow. Other approaches may be available to us which may be important steps toward improving the dementia experience.

Luckily, we don't have to start from scratch. There are ways of examining how networks and communities are influenced by change and challenges that can be helpful in rethinking dementia. This book will describe a new way of considering dementia utilising "systems thinking", the notion that many aspects of our world are shaped by the interaction of and change within complex systems. These systems can be of many types and those affecting dementia include but are not limited to the systems of ideas we use to understand dementia as a society; the social and relational systems of those around and providing care for a person with dementia; and the interaction of personal psychological, spiritual, cognitive and physical systems for a person with dementia. These all play a part in creating "dementia". Dementia, as a biological process of changing neuronal structures and pathways, directly affects some of these systems but these changes also have effects that ripple outwards to contribute to a larger and more complicated systemic notion of "dementia".

It is worth restating that dementia is a process involving continual change. The sorts of observed changes that are often associated with dementia, particularly those of memory, language, decision-making, behaviour and relationships have important implications for key parts of what people value about their lives. How these changes intersect with values such as identity, autonomy and personhood are important and will be explored further throughout this book. Additionally, we will explore the relationships between the direct changes caused by dementia and the changes in the systems that are impacted by this syndrome. The social systems of dementia networks (the communities of people, including the person with dementia themselves, and those who are closest to a person with dementia) tend to be influenced (perturbed) by certain types of changes. The network's response to these changes can lead to either a more robust and stable network, or a network that becomes more fragmented. Understanding why this happens, and what brings about changes in these networks may be critical in better supporting people with dementia and their networks.

Hopefully, you are feeling reassured at this point that this book might have something in it for you. It may be that you're more interested in some parts of what we're going to explore than others. To make it a little easier to figure out how to make your way through the book, I'll provide some additional information about each part and whom it might interest.

• • •

PART ONE of the book is called "The weight of dementia". It explores what dementia is as an illness, but it also starts to unpack the many things that dementia means to us and why they make the problem even harder to deal with. The history of the idea of "dementia" is an important focus in early sections. This early part of the book provides context for later ideas and won't be a bad place to start for most readers. Philosophical ideas (like autonomy, identity and personhood) which have had a big impact on what dementia means are covered in some depth in the later part of this section. If you are interested in philosophy, ethics or the implications of these challenges for people with dementia (how we decide how valuable a person with dementia's experience or life is, for example), you'll get a lot out of this section. Or you may decide to skip this section. It will all be waiting here for you if you decide to check in again later. This part of the book finishes with an interlude chapter about the sorts of things that you need to keep in mind if you want to do research involving people with dementia. This interlude section will certainly interest people with questions about how research is done with and for people with dementia.

PART TWO of the book, "Dementia's impact and ripples" moves away from focusing primarily on what we can learn from reading about dementia and the ideas that affect what it means. This part of the book is focused on what people with dementia, the family members and friends who care for them and the people who work in dementia care (dementia networks), say about their experiences. It is divided into chapters that address key themes of what the people I have spoken to about their experiences revealed. They revealed that dementia isn't one thing but a complex of different experiences and expectations and there's a chapter ("The dementia manifold") which shares examples of what they said and digs into what this might mean. If you are interested in what other people have said about what dementia feels like this is probably a good chapter for you. Members of dementia networks also talked about decision-making in dementia. Decisions aren't simple either, there's a lot involved in making them and they have a momentum which creates and commits us to a path forward. The chapter "Decisions in dementia: stepping stones in the river" explores these ideas and what other thinkers have said which can help us make sense of them. People who are interested in how decision-making tends to happen in dementia should get a lot out of this chapter. The final chapter in this part is "Our, not your, dementia". This chapter reveals the impact of dementia on relationships, what is challenged, what is nurtured and what this can help us learn about dementia. People with an interest in what dementia means for relationships will find this a really useful chapter.

PART THREE, "From networks to systems", is where some new thinking starts. These chapters begin by helping us get up to speed with what systems theory means and how systems thinking might apply to our understanding the dementia experience. The first two chapters are probably going to be useful to anyone unfamiliar with systems thinking and who wants to understand the key ideas of this book. The second chapter, "Systems in dementia" provides some explanation of how I've used these ideas about systems to try to understand what I've heard from dementia networks. This chapter is probably going to be important for anyone who wants to understand the final chapter of this part, "Making sense of change", which explores stories of dementia networks, revealing that there's more we can pick up if we're paying the right kind of attention. For those wanting to read more about the lived experiences of the networks of people affected by dementia, this section has the most concentrated collection of their stories. It will be of interest for anyone who wants to understand the implications of this book or who just wants to read more about what the dementia experience can be like for those who are immersed in it.

PART FOUR, "Rethinking dementia", brings the other parts of the book together. It outlines what we've discovered and what it might mean for us all when we're working together to support people with dementia as best we can into the future. This part also includes some humbly offered words of advice that may have some resonance for you. This part should be of interest to anyone who's found other parts of the book interesting. However, if you want to know the answers that I've found (or at least the next set of questions that I've identified) through my work with dementia to date, then feel free to skip forward to this final section.

The ideas in this book have arisen from research work with people with dementia and dementia networks that also include the person's families, friends, carers and clinicians. Their stories are part of the evidence to support the ideas developed in this research and will also be used to explain and explore key points. These stories, and the ideas in this book, are not a complete exploration of all that can occur in dementia, but they hold important insights to ensure that we are learning from dementia and improving our responses to it. In effect, this book suggests that we shouldn't just wait for a medical advance to "cure" dementia, but that we should do all that we can to live with and learn from dementia for as long as we need to.

Acknowledgments

I'd like to acknowledge the tremendous support that I've had at all stages in turning this area of my life from a conversation with colleagues to something which I hope has and will be meaningful to many. To begin with, I'd like to thank my colleagues and mentors Professor Paul Komesaroff and Professor Jenny Philip. Paul and Jenny, for all the support you've given as guides on my steps to date, for all the inspiration and enthusiasm, for encouraging my abiding interest in the human, the complex and the unanswerable, for being astounding objects of admiration, for your deeply treasured friendship, and for your peerless warmth and kindness, I thank you.

To the people with dementia, their carers and their healthcare providers who have helped kindle and nurture the ideas in this book, you have been so amazingly generous with the stories and experiences that have taught me so much. I can only hope to be able to honour and repay you in some small way through work like this. I thank you.

To the marvellous contributors and collaborators who have contributed to this work in too many ways to document, including Dr Elissa Campbell, Dr Nathan D'Cunha, Professor Deborah Clark, Professor Deborah Parker, Professor Aileen Collier, Professor Martin Fuchs, Professor Steven Sabat, Professor Ian Kerridge, Professor Lucy Burke, Professor Pia Kontos, and Kai Ping Tan, I thank you for support, for your ideas, for your energy, and for your passion. To Mirranda Burton, I feel so lucky to have been able to work with you on this book and to share your inspirational vision and art. To Dr Sally Gardner at Palaver, thank you for the work you've put into making this book look like it was written by someone more skilled than me. To my friends and family who've kindly read this book and helped it become what it is, including Gloria Armellin and Rowan Wyborn, I thank you.

To my family who've been patient and semi-willing participants in the efforts and focus that this work has involved, who've tolerated me and my late nights, and who I love and adore beyond words, I thank you. To Bree, my partner in all things, I can never adequately express my thanks and my love. To Ernie, who has never known a time when I wasn't working on this book in some form, I hope that this and more of what my generation does helps make your time on this earth a little better. To Mitzie, my proof-poodle, you got us there.

PART ONE

The weight of dementia

1. Understanding the weight of dementia

A diagnosis of dementia means something. It has a weight to it. Returning to the metaphor of the stone dropped into a pool, receiving the news, the actuality of dementia is heavy and dense. It has an enormous impact. While this is true, a lot of things believed about dementia are probably not true qualities of the stone but extra things that are cobbled on to it. In effect, it may be that we make the stone of dementia bigger and heavier than it needs to be, and its impact increases accordingly.

There are a lot of good reasons why we do this. Some are so fundamental to the way we live that we barely notice them. There are some key things about who we feel we are and what we value about ourselves that dementia seems to threaten in profound ways. Many of us have always lived in societies in which personal independence and autonomy (the quality of self-rule) are intrinsically associated with what it means to live a valuable life. The importance of our ability to be independent and autonomous, therefore, makes sense to us and the idea of losing our independence is one of the things that we all find quietly terrifying. Dementia is almost perfectly targeted at this knot of self-worry, this anxiety about whether we will be able to maintain our individuality and "me-ness" and continue to determine who we are and what we will do next. How could we not fear it?

But what if these worries aren't as solid as they seem? What if the much-vaunted importance of our autonomy and independence wasn't actually as solid, as helpful or as real as we might believe? What if there's more value to dementia than we think, and more to value in people who have dementia than is often obvious? What if the stone of dementia is, to some extent, a weight of our own making? This part of the book will start to work through some of these questions and ideas so we can start to get to the bottom of what dementia is, and why it has such an impact on us.

2. What is dementia to us?

Let me share another story.

When I met Nancy for the first time in the care facility where she lived, her friend and carer, Rosie, was keen to be there. It's not unusual for families and friends to want to help support a person with dementia when they meet someone new, particularly when that someone is a healthcare professional. I assumed that was why Rosie wanted to be there. Almost as soon as I met Nancy, I decided that I was wrong. Rosie wasn't there to help Nancy, she was there to help me not get shoo-ed out of the door as soon as I arrived.

Nancy was a strong person. She was tough, and she was clever. She had the brusqueness of someone who'd had a lifetime of more important things to do than she'd had moments to spare. From an early age she'd been "farmed out" to others by her family in regional Victoria. Her family was poor, and her father was never able to hold down a job after returning from the war. There were too many mouths at home to feed reliably. Nancy had also learned her independence early and thoroughly. As a child she was creative and clever. She was quick to question and point out inconsistencies, a trait which often inspired adults around her to take action to control this uppity young girl. Her parents felt that sending her away made sense on multiple levels.

As a young adult she moved to the city and discovered her passion for caring through training as a nurse. She felt a real bond with the destitute and the "dead-beats" in her care in the religious city hospital. Her patients appreciated her kindness, and she felt a kinship with them that she didn't feel with the "stuffy nuns" who ran the hospital. She moved back to the land and continued nursing, but the move re-kindled her deep love for the Australian bush. She became an artist and conservationist. She treasured the bush and her animal friends and took a personal and sometimes painful stand against anything she felt threatened them.

Nancy attracted others. Her passion, her generosity, and her eccentricity drew people in. She was surrounded by people, but also kept them at a distance. She had only a few close friends who were obviously devoted to her, and fairly limited contact with her brothers and sisters. Kerrie, her General Practitioner (GP), wondered whether this combination of Nancy's strong identity, and the fact that none of the broad group of people around her knew her that well or were very involved in her life might have had an impact on how late it was that some of her difficulties were picked up. Nancy forgot things but was dismissive about their importance. Losing track of who had her paintings didn't matter to her because her joy in them was in the painting. Not remembering to have meals didn't matter because she's always been thin and wiry. Her grand old house had become tattered, but she would sagely remind others that she'd lived in far worse. Nancy felt her lapses were more real and worrying when it became clear she could no longer take care of the native animals she sheltered. Risking their well-being was intolerable and, for Nancy, meant that something was going wrong. It was only later that she learned that this was due to dementia.

My meeting with Nancy and Rosie was five years later, by which time a lot more had changed. Nancy shared her views on her life, talking about what she'd loved and what she'd lost. She told me a story about a lifelong friend, Victoria, with whom she'd recently had a terrible falling out. Smiling, Nancy told me that eventually they'd made up and remained close friends to this day. It was at that point that Rosie, hesitantly, told us that Victoria had died of a heart attack a few months ago. I wasn't expecting this sad twist, and, as I watched, I realised that Nancy who had lived through every moment of this story was clearly floored by the news. Nancy was sad and quiet but recovered quickly. It felt like this turn of events, the sudden and shocking news of the death of Nancy's friend of many years, was also not that surprising as she sat with it and tested it out for herself. She'd lost the content of the story but some sense of the shape of it remained, like an empty picture frame hanging on a familiar wall. A frame which suddenly became crowded with colour and meaning as the details of her story were shared once more.

Nancy had dementia. "Dementia" has a lot of meanings. Most simply, dementia means a progressive change in how our central nervous tissues (particularly parts of our brain) function and communicate with each other (a neurodegenerative syndrome) which is more common with increasing age. Dementia can involve a constellation of changes or symptoms, including changes in our use of language, our executive function (the planning, focusing, task-juggling, decision-making parts of how we think), memory, and behaviour. When these abilities are affected by dementia, changes tend to progress over months and years. In Nancy's story we can see reference to many of these kinds of changes, but it's also clear to me as a doctor, a researcher and a person, that dementia must be more than this. When I was in medical school, I remember learning that the commonest feature of dementia is memory loss. But, even if that's true, it's clearly a woeful simplification of something much more complex. Saying that dementia often involves memory loss doesn't come close to expressing what it must be like for people like Nancy and Rosie to share a moment when Nancy realises that she has forgotten that an incredibly important person in her life has died. To this day, I'm not sure whether it is Nancy's forgetting or how quickly this information became real for her that moves me so deeply when I think about these moments with her. The death of her friend seemed completely inaccessible to Nancy even while it had marked her in some deep way that remained familiar to her. It was only after I thanked Nancy and Rosie for their generosity and their time and was travelling home that I realised that that moment wouldn't have happened if Rosie and I hadn't been there, talking about Victoria. Nancy's experiences were so clearly tied up with what others did and said.

We'll come back to this point multiple times, but I think it's clear that dementia is a complex idea without a single specific meaning. But perhaps a good way to start mapping out all the things that dementia might mean is to explore some of the clearest contributors to it. When people say "dementia" they are often talking about Alzheimer's disease. Dementia and Alzheimer's disease are not the same thing, but they're often terms that are used interchangeably when we talk about these sorts of problems. Medically speaking, Alzheimer's disease is the most common and most studied illness contributing to dementia but there are many other potential causes (McKhann et al., 2011). A common approach to diagnosing dementia (according to the American *Diagnostic and Statistical Manual* or DSM, edition V) describes it as present when a person has a significant decline in one or more areas of their cognition where these changes interfere with their ability to be independent in the way they want or used to be and where these problems aren't better explained by another cause (Sachdev et al., 2014). These areas of cognition are: complex attention (a person's ability to sustain, divide and select their attention); executive ability (a person's ability to plan, decide, be mentally flexible, respond to feedback, use their working memory); learning and memory (a person's immediate, recent and long term memory); language (a person's ability to express and understand language); visual-motor perception (a person's ability to perform familiar tasks and orientate themselves); and social cognition (a person's ability to recognise emotion, regulate their behaviour and manage social expectations). A person with an Alzheimer's type of dementia is more likely to have earlier problems with learning and memory often alongside subtle changes in executive ability, language and visual-motor perception (Apostolova, 2016). Other types of dementia can start with different types of early features. Generally speaking, as dementia becomes more advanced there are more symptoms involving more areas of cognition, and differentiating types of dementia becomes more difficult. Simply put, the longer a person has dementia, the subtle cues that help us figure out what the cause might be are harder and harder to pick up. It's also important to note that newer approaches to assessment can mean that a person could be diagnosed with pathological brain changes consistent with Alzheimer's disease without actually having a dementia syndrome (as we discussed above). This is something we'll discuss a bit later on as it's a developing and complicated area. However, overall, this means that a person with dementia doesn't necessarily have Alzheimer's disease, and a person with Alzheimer's disease doesn't necessarily have dementia.

Our focus in this book is exploring dementia more generally, rather than spending too much time focusing on the different types. Early in the book we're going to talk more about Alzheimer's disease, as our focus in these early sections is understanding what's been thought and written about dementia; and Alzheimer's disease is the condition which has had the lion's share of the attention. As the book progresses, our language will shift and the focus will be more on dementia as a single if large and complicated idea. This is because many of the challenges and experiences that we'll explore aren't really related to the specific causes of dementia for people, but seem to be more related to dementia itself. Obviously, this may not always be true in all situations, but it seems true for the issues we're going to talk through in this book.

Both dementia and Alzheimer's disease are ideas that have become more prominent over time. It's true that there are more people who have dementia around now, both because we're better at recognising dementia due to our more sophisticated medical assessments, and because we are living longer, and dementia is more common as we age. But there's more to dementia's prominence than this. We're deeply aware of dementia and affected by it as a community, not just because many people have dementia but also because we're tuned to consider this phenomenon as important. A variety of historical and cultural influences have resulted in dementia becoming an idea which grabs our attention and often worries us deeply. A central influence is probably the ways that we, and those who have come before us, have viewed and understood what we value about ourselves and how we understand disability, dependence, and vulnerability in our societies.

Human cultures have grappled with the concept of dementia for longer than many of us would assume. The ancient Egyptians described cognitive impairment in their writings, and the idea of dementia itself can be traced back to the ancient Greeks (George et al., 2011). It's fascinating that a focus of these early references to dementia was its social implications, such as its impact on a person's right and ability to make decisions for themselves (in a civil or legal sense). Ancient responses seemed less troubled by why dementia happened or what it was, and more on how people who had these sorts of problems should be treated. There were rules about the rights and responsibilities of a person with dementia. For example, that they weren't permitted to sign a testamentary will or couldn't be charged with committing a crime (Kurz & Lautenschlager, 2009). These early ideas about dementia unveil our millennia of grappling with questions that remain central today, namely: how should people with dementia fit within society; how should they be listened to; and how should we respond to decisions that people with dementia make or need to make?

The word "dementia" itself (literally "away" or "out" of "mind" or "reason" in Latin) entered the English language from the French *démence* via psychiatrist Phillipe Pinel in the late 18th century (George et al., 2011). Around this time, there was an increasing focus on classifying diseases into scientific categories or taxonomies. This new scientific understanding recognised diseases as occurring because of things which affected structures within the body and mind. "Dementia" was accepted as a medical concept within this developing approach to understanding illness (George et al., 2011). Dementia was believed to occur because of discrete and observable neuropathological changes within the substance of the brain. That is, dementia was understood as an "organic" disease of an individual person, a change which could be explained by finding and pointing out a specific problem (Kurz & Lautenschlager, 2009).

Against this background, Alzheimer's disease was initially described by Alois Alzheimer prior to Emil Kraepelin publishing a pathological definition in 1910. At this early point, these clinicians had identified a group of people who shared similar and ongoing changes in their thinking, communication and behaviour. Further examination of these people after they died showed that they also had similar microscopic changes in their brains when their brain samples were examined under a microscope. In combination, these observations suggested a single medical problem which was given the name Alzheimer's disease. At that point, it wasn't clear why and how these behavioural and anatomical things were linked, and thus that there was little prospect of progress on a treatment for Alzheimer's disease. However, even without a medical treatment, care practices for people with Alzheimer's were developed. People with the diagnosis needed help with the impacts of dementia. Early dementia management relied mainly on a non-medical, often a psychological or social focus, approach to understanding the illness and providing care and support (George et al., 2011), elements which remain centrally important today.

This focus on social and psychological responses to dementia changed radically in the 1970s, along with a significant shift towards a more contemporary medical search for dementia treatments. New scientific techniques and assessments, including advances in the imaging and microscopic studies of the brain, gave hope that a clear neuropathological cause for dementia, and therefore new techniques to respond to it, was within reach (Whitehouse, 1985). It seems safe to say now that this early optimism was a little premature. In this period, the brain changes that seemed to cause dementia could be detected clearly, but understanding how these related to the experience of the condition was a point of conjecture. Nonetheless, Alzheimer's disease, as a solid and clear diagnosis, emerged from a process of study, attention and advocacy mainly in the United States, triggering a variety of social changes that we continue to live with and through.

Many advances have taken place since that time, including a more complete understanding of the role of classic brain changes in Alzheimer's disease known as "amyloid plaques", "neurofibrillary tangles" and "'neuritic plaques". A key result has been the view that the proliferation of amyloid plaque in the human brain (the so-called "amyloid cascade hypothesis") is central to the development of Alzheimer's disease (Panza et al., 2019). Controversy continues in some areas despite our progress. Experts are divided on some issues, such as which of the detectable changes in Alzheimer's disease we should be trying to fix. We've also come to understand that increasing age is often associated with a variety of brain changes in people with dementia which may or may not be causing problems, complicating our hopes for a simple fix (Schneider et al., 2009). So, despite our sophisticated understanding of pathologies, there's a lot we still don't know or don't understand. For example, we aren't sure why some people may have pathological features of Alzheimer's disease on some tests but don't have dementia, and others with clinical features of dementia don't have the expected pathological findings (Deture & Dickson, 2019). It seems likely (but perhaps not surprising) that dementia is more complicated than we took it for. For instance, what we call Alzheimer's disease may be a syndrome, a collection of things which look similar, rather than a singular problem with one cause. Alzheimer's disease as we usually understand it probably results from multiple types of brain changes, for multiple reasons and related to multiple risk factors over the course of a lifetime (Richards & Brayne, 2010). This notion is supported by findings from neuropathological studies suggesting that most people whom we would expect to have "Alzheimer's disease" as a cause for their dementia changes actually have a variety of different types of changes in their brain which aren't usually considered as components of this pathology (Deture & Dickson, 2019). Some studies suggest that modern medicine hasn't been able to determine a single cause or way of preventing Alzheimer's disease or made clear how it is different from ageing (Plassman et al., 2010). This suggests that, rather than being clear and tightly defined problems, Alzheimer's and dementia might be part of a continuum of neurocognitive changes from a variety of different causes all of which are more common as we grow older (George et al., 2011).

With this background, it's probably less of a surprise that our pathological knowledge of dementia hasn't yet translated into much impact on the process of diagnosing dementia or knowing what it might mean for a person in the future. Some exciting developments have occurred, such as in the advent of biomarkers for dementia. These are tests, often imaging studies such as PET or MRI, or examinations of the cerebral spinal fluid, which can support the clinical diagnosis of dementia by indirectly assessing pathological changes in the brain without needing to resort to looking at brain tissue under a microscope. These approaches seem promising, but their current cost and complexity mean that they are of limited use or unavailable for most people (Fink et al., 2020). For most people diagnosed with dementia, the process to get there hasn't changed much in decades. A diagnosis of dementia usually results from a clinician (often a specialist doctor) taking a history, doing a clinical examination and using bedside tools like questionnaires, assessing a person's language, their memory, how they behave and react and the impact of any of these types of changes on how they live in society.

It is also unfortunately true that our progress towards being able to slow, halt or reverse dementia has been limited. Virtually all (99.6%) medical treatments intended to affect the accepted neuropathological contributors to Alzheimer's disease over the decade from 2002 to 2012 failed to establish the evidence required for routine clinical use (Cummings et al., 2014). Over twenty-five randomised controlled trials seeking to test the validity of the amyloid cascade hypothesis by trying to disrupt this process have led to negative results, leading some to call for a fundamental re-consideration of what changes are truly pathological in Alzheimer dementia (Alexander et al., 2021; Panza et al., 2019). The challenges of treating Alzheimer's disease have become even more clear due to a recent qualified success story. The first new medication therapy for Alzheimer's disease was approved by the Food and Drug Administration (FDA) in the USA (aducanumab, a human monoclonal antibody targeting Beta amyloid fibrils and oligomers) in 2021. However, this occurred under controversial circumstances and with arguable evidence to support its approval and its routine use (Alexander et al., 2021). Defending their decision for the approval of aducanumab without the usual supportive evidence, the FDA described being moved to act by the "devastating toll" of Alzheimer's and citing many patients and families who made clear that they would rather accept the uncertainty of benefit and the risks of novel treatments than the feared decline of dementia (Dunn et al., 2021). Our options to treat Alzheimer's remain limited but our desperation to do so continues to climb.

While it is clearly a tragic predicament, many of us wouldn't be surprised by the idea that people would accept many known and unknown risks for a possible chance at improving or stopping dementia. Studies have shown us that people wish to avoid Alzheimer's disease no matter the cost and report being willing to accept a 30% chance of death or permanent disability from a hypothetical drug to limit the progression of mild dementia (Hauber et al., 2009). The idea of dementia is deeply threatening to us. In Australia, my home country, dementia is feared second only to cancer, and it is arguable whether cancer will remain the "winner" given the new optimism surrounding modern cancer treatments (Phillipson et al., 2012). Many of us would choose any state or fate over having dementia. In the 1990s, older adults and persons in care facilities, that is, people who don't have dementia, rated the idea of having dementia as a state "worse than death" and there's little evidence to suggest this judgement has changed (Patrick et al., 1994). This probably isn't a result of more people being exposed to dementia and determining a view on this experience. While dementia is becoming more common, people in many communities now have less exposure to ageing and its challenges than used to be the case. It used to be common for family units to provide care to older people in many cultures and countries, but now care of older generations increasingly relies on institutional facilities. Many of us don't see people with dementia and, so, our fear of it cannot be explained by direct experience. But we clearly have strong feelings about the idea of dementia. We feel that having dementia would mark and change us in fundamental ways. Population studies show us that people anticipate that being diagnosed with dementia would lead to shame, fear and depression, and be a source of stigma (Phillipson et al., 2012). Our responses to dementia permeate the spaces around it, affecting us prior to us ever encountering it.

Old fears in new clothes

People anticipate and fear the experience of dementia for many reasons. Some common, understandable and fairly obvious reasons are that it is common, it is progressive, that it affects how we think, communicate and act, and that there aren't effective treatments for it. But there's more to our fear of dementia than this. To begin to understand why we fear dementia we need to explore what dementia means beyond being a medical diagnosis. Dementia is encased by layers of cultural meaning, a thick cocoon of expectations, beliefs, and stories that influence how we talk and think about it. At the same time, how we talk and think about dementia adds to these layers, often resulting in a self-fulfilling narrative where we see and experience what we expect to find.

Dementia has not always been feared everywhere and to this extent its meanings shift and change. Our common current negative expectations, however, have a real impact on those with dementia and those involved in caring for them.

The language that we use for dementia is a good barometer for gauging what we think about it. Written descriptions, such as on the internet or in media, often focus on how dementia leads to the loss of important human qualities. Alzheimer's and dementia are described as being hopeless conditions which rob us of our selves, leaving nothing behind that we'd recognise as us, or even as a human being. Usual descriptions of dementia in the media include "the assassin of the mind", "the long goodbye", "the silent epidemic", with Alzheimer's as a disease which "steals the mind", and "makes shells of our former selves" (Smith, 2009). Dementia is a "funeral without end" (Herskovits, 1995). Through our words, dementia has been given the power to metaphorically transform us into non-humans. People are described as descending into animals, lower forms of life such as dogs or primates without human-like capacities (Degrazia, 2005; Pierce, 2000). Our words also conjure deeper descents into the realm of the monstrous, where the victims of the condition are zombies in a state of living death (Behuniak, 2011). It is not just the change in the individual that is monstrous but the relentless and primordial power of dementia itself (Chapman et al., 2018). In *Still Alice* by Lisa Genova, the main character and narrator, Alice, who has been diagnosed with Alzheimer's disease, rails against her dementia wishing it were cancer so that some fight would be possible. But Alice sees dementia as an overwhelming natural force, a beast with "no weapons that could slay it" (Genova, 2009: 86). For her, it is the "unstoppable, ferocious, destructive" force of the ocean dragging the self away into its depths. The depths here are places of the lost, such as those described in Jonathan Franzen's *The Corrections*, where dementia is a "darkness" that consumes the person even as they try to escape (Franzen, 2010).

It's important to note that the emotive and powerful language we use when we describe dementia is not accidental. There are reasons why dementia is framed in this way, and in some cases the language was chosen in the hope of promoting specific outcomes. Most notably descriptions of dementia have been intended primarily to guide or shape public thinking. In the 1970s, dementia began to be recognised as an issue that required social and cultural attention. Populations were ageing and additional challenges were on the horizon. Dementia became a focus and communicative vehicle for these concerns. Clinicians, researchers, and interest groups consciously used this opportune concern to harness additional attention, resources, and funding (George, 2010). Some of our language for dementia, rhetorical devices seeking to influence community discussions and expressing a need for urgent responses, may have their roots here. One approach has been to use the language of disaster to describe the momentum and volume of dementia cases or care needs. Descriptions of the dementia "epidemic", "the rising tide" or "the silent tsunami" convey an impression that dementia is a colossal and unstoppable force. Dementia is, as we've discussed, becoming more common primarily because there are more of us who are living longer and dementia is more common with ageing, but that (fairly dry) explanation doesn't fit the power dementia seems to have within media descriptions. The language used describes our response to dementia as heroic resistance against impossible odds. It's not too many steps further to personify the force of dementia as actually intending us harm. Dementia doesn't just affect us, in many writer's hands it is a "deadly" killer (Brookes et al., 2018). Now, it is important to acknowledge that dementia is a progressive condition currently without a cure, and it is a common and increasing cause or contributor to dying for many people. However, reporting on these points is often focused — far more emotively — on a violent dementia causing more deaths, rather than on the more truthful sense that we're successfully living long enough for dementia to cause us more problems and are now better at detecting and diagnosing dementia when it's present. Appreciating dementia as an inescapable killer seems to suggest that we need an equally powerful and violent response to its evil intent (Zeilig, 2014). Thus, military metaphors to describe response to dementia are common within the scientific literature, in advocacy campaigns, and in the general media (Lane et al., 2013). Dementia response campaign titles such as, "Developing the framework for an international battle against Alzheimer's Disease" and the "War on Alzheimer's Disease" are representative of a general call to arms to beat back dementia (Gleckman, 2012; Rosow et al., 2011). We spend so much time focusing on the power of dementia and the need for others to engage with the problems it creates that sometimes the people most affected by it, the people who actually have dementia, seem to be left out. The images we use when we're talking about dementia highlight this. Pictures of sad and lost looking older people with dementia being comforted by others, or people with dementia being represented by more abstract images like pictures of hands, make people with dementia seem passive and less important to the dementia story, as merely background characters to what is occurring (Brookes et al., 2018). These images, combined with the language choices noted above, suggest that what's needed is for all the well people to stand up to dementia, rather than for more to be done to understand what's happening for those who are actually affected by it.

The choices we make when we describe dementia have an impact and reveal much about what dementia means to us. It's clearly valuable for us to talk publicly about dementia, to focus on its impact and use a shared and readily understood approach to describing it. Emotive descriptions demand attention and can motivate people to think and act differently. Some of the language noted above is clearly intended to help people understand that we need to think and talk more about dementia, providing impetus for additional community attention and resourcing (Lane et al., 2013). However, these metaphors may also limit our considering and managing the problems associated with dementia in other ways, effectively stopping us from seeing dementia, or those with dementia, in any other way (George & Whitehouse, 2014).

Declaring "war" on dementia positions people with that condition as passive victims in the battle being fought on their behalf. This, of course, highlights their need for support but also unintentionally diminishes the meaningfulness of their role or their potential to do anything without our help. It suggests that dementia experiences become valid and important because of the support that they receive. Focusing on "fighting" dementia, and the accumulation of new pharmaceutical weapons to do so, may inadvertently diminish our focus on caring for persons with this incurable condition and may complicate planning for their future declining health (Lane et al., 2013). As described above, in the relatively recent example of the FDA approval of aducanumab, choosing to view dementia as a fight at all costs influences how we think about the next steps to take and how to balance risks and benefits. Largely untested or unproven "wartime" strategies in dementia care, such as treatments or pre-symptomatic screening, can be seen as necessary for victory, even if the consequences of their use aren't fully understood (Couteur et al., 2013).

It's important to know that this isn't just about representations of dementia in the media. These language choices, and their impact, go all the way down, having powerful and pervasive effects on how people relate to and understand each other. Understanding dementia as an evil enemy to be overcome, and a person with dementia as a victim to be saved, naturally encourages us to focus on rescuing people with dementia. Wishing to win that war doesn't make us bad people. But seeing situations through a lens can colour what we perceive. There's a saying that, "if you have a hammer everything looks like a nail".[1] In this situation because we "know" that dementia must be fixed, when we see people with dementia we see only victims, not people. This has implications for clinical relationships, too, where care choices (between doctors, nurses, clinicians, care workers, patients and families) are influenced by preconceptions in language. Language and metaphors describing illness and treatments can shape what we consider as normal clinical practice over time and what sorts of care options are considered appropriate, are offered and are provided (Bleakley et al., 2014). It is not difficult to see why clinicians, patients and families are drawn toward the metaphoric light and hope of potential treatment in contrast to the darkness and shadow of dementia (Zeilig, 2014).

While there is some contemporary evidence that the tone and quality of media reporting on dementia may have improved, negative perceptions of dementia continue to have a cultural impact (Doyle et al., 2012). The meaning of dementia is assumed to be "disaster", and the term "dementia" itself is now considered as substitutable (a metonym) for doom, dependence, and decline (Zeilig, 2014). This means that we've moved beyond just the impact of the words we use when we're describing dementia. The idea of dementia has cultural expectations deeply tied to it, and these have an impact on our expectations of dementia, our response to the experiences of those who have it, and, tragically, society's ability to manage the condition. These expressions, stories and stereotypes have the effect of distancing "us", the "normal" people without dementia, from "them", the abnormal, embarrassing, feared and somewhat monstrous quasi-people with dementia (Zeilig, 2014). It changes the rules, so that what might be appropriate, beneficial and permissible for us seems a little bit different for them. As much as we might wish otherwise, we all will, at some point, be more frail, more dependent on others, and be close to dying. It may be that some of the reasons that we respond so negatively to dementia is because it reminds us of these uncomfortable truths that we'd rather ignore for as long as possible. Dementia seems to be a part of what has been described as the "abject", inescapable aspects of ourselves that we repulse and reject, because they simultaneously seem meaningless and deeply significant (Kristeva, 1982). We might be fighting so hard to ignore and cast away dementia because it is so important, and because our worries about it are so universal. In warring against dementia, we're ultimately then wounding ourselves, as it may be through dementia that we have the best lesson about our inescapable human frailty and vulnerability (George & Whitehouse, 2014).

Whilst our use of language may explain some of the fear that Alzheimer's disease raises in our community, it does not explain it all. Dementia and Alzheimer's disease represent fears that we already nurse as individuals and as a society, they are a visible focus and representation of these concerns rather than being their source. The "descent of Alzheimer's disease contributes to the story we tell ourselves about ourselves" as we grapple with the idea of becoming old, and being less than we were (Herskovits, 1995). Why do we think getting older means becoming less than we used to be? It's a fascinating and important question. At least one part of the answer is our society's focus on youth and the importance of ideas like individualism (being independent and self-reliant) and rationality (being led by logic and reason). We tend to view ourselves as independent beings, as "unified, coherent and rational agent(s)" who are the authors of our "own experience and meaning", a type of thinking which is often termed "humanism" (Burr, 1995). But this "humanistic" focus, where we prize being independent and rational, seems to suggest that people who need more help and are less clearly rational, people with dementia, for example, are less "normal" and ultimately less than human. Understanding how this perception may have evolved requires us to explore a key idea that has been important and influential since the Renaissance (the modern era), and core to the problem of how we understand dementia, namely, the concept of "personal autonomy".

3. Autonomy: a rambling citadel

The idea of autonomy has been central in describing what we value about ourselves. It is, like dementia, an old idea which has become even more relevant to people in the last few hundred years. As we'll discuss, these two ideas — autonomy and dementia — are important foils for each other, with the importance of autonomy and the worry about its loss being pivotal in how concerned we are about things — like dementia — that seem to threaten it.

The modern concept of autonomy

The core element of "autonomy" is the capacity for self-governance, being able to do what is needed without external influence or control. This idea is built into the word itself, as a combination of Ancient Greek *autos* (self) and *nomos* (rule or law). Autonomy does not only apply to individual people: a state may be autonomous from another state even if both are closely connected, such as the Vatican City and Italy. Early use of the word focused on just this point, with Greek city states having *autonomia* when they made their own laws independent of outside control. From these political roots it slowly became clear that a more personal sense of autonomy was also very important (Ashley, 2012). But this development has been long and complicated. Even if the idea of a person governing themselves seems simple superficially, it soon gets complicated. It has been suggested that we can make the idea manageable by breaking autonomy down into four different but important things: the capacity or ability to govern ourselves (being able to be autonomous), actually doing or achieving this (being autonomous), an ideal that we find important that we might aspire to (wanting autonomy), and as a right or set of rights which expresses our self-governance (having a right to autonomy) (J. Feinberg, 1989).

In this chapter we'll touch on all these facets of autonomy in our efforts to understand the implications for dementia. To make a small start on that let's consider another story:

> The first time I met Tim and Ellen, Tim made a shrewd observation. We were talking about how things change. They'd just finished telling me about how they hoped that their new mini schnauzer (Oscar), who seemed trenchantly impervious to attempts to let him know what a "good dog" would do, would start to become more like

their old, recently departed and terribly missed dog. Tim noted that a lot had changed for them beyond Oscar's arrival. For Tim, a lot of this was related to what he or others thought he could or should do. He remarked, "Well, you are probably not the best judge of your own abilities, but I still feel within myself that I am capable of doing what I have always done."

Tim had been diagnosed with dementia three years previously. Doctors and other professionals had suggested that this should have all sorts of implications for Tim, but he wasn't as certain. He was happy to hear from "the experts" but felt confident about what was best for him and felt that he "could probably do a bit more than some other people gave (him) credit for". A major challenge was when the experts suggested he should restrict his driving. Tim loved the "daring, the danger and the spectacle" of motor sports. He'd always felt comfortable around cars. More than that, the mechanical reliability of a good engine led to an ease in Tim. He felt relaxed and in control when he was behind the wheel. His doctor suggested he drive less and for shorter distances. She told him that he could take a medical driving test but discouraged this as she felt that he'd likely lose his licence all together. This felt like a huge risk for Tim. The idea of never driving again was a considerable threat. Tim worried about an emergency when he might need to drive, to "step up and take charge" as he'd always done. Continuing to drive and the freedom it gave him held an importance that he wouldn't easily give up.

Ellen was privately unsure that they'd struck the right balance with Tim's driving. Tim would go out for drives by himself and was always cagey about whether he'd been sticking to the limits set out by the doctor. She was also sure that asking Tim to "step up" in a crisis wasn't realistic or fair. He'd needed to do that before, and it hadn't gone well. A year ago, Ellen had slipped on a patch of ice, fallen and broken her knee cap. In that moment of crisis Tim hadn't known what to do and Ellen was initially too distressed to help. He kept getting confused and insisting that she walk when she couldn't. He hadn't been able to follow the ambulance to the hospital in his car and they'd ended up needing to get help from friends to retrieve it. Despite the pain, Ellen had felt the biggest challenge of the day had been keeping Tim calm and safe while she was being assessed in hospital.

Ellen had learned to be cautious about expressing any opinion that disagreed with his. She'd suggested that they should get someone else to cut down a tree in their backyard, and Tim had become angry at her for implying that he couldn't do it. "You're just being negative," he would say and accuse her of undercutting him. What she'd meant, she felt, was that she was worried that it wasn't safe, but she didn't know how to convey this to him. It seemed that all he could hear was criticism, or worse, a sense that he didn't have as much to contribute to their lives anymore.

Ellen's response was to try to find a balance by encouraging Tim to do what she felt he could do, to give him more self-confidence. But these moments of conflict led to revelation. Ellen eventually realised that she could work around Tim without him knowing. If Tim did a task badly, she'd quietly fix it with no one the wiser. Resolving their long-term pitched battles about Tim's collecting items like stationery and packaging "just in case they're needed" was also, she realised, as easy as throwing things away and never mentioning it. Tim's amnesia had provided a powerful tool that she used liberally. If Tim got angry, Ellen felt that there was no longer any point trying to reason with him, so she'd just walk away. If she did this, she realised, she would win and he would settle down, because she would be the only one who remembered. Tim's memory loss had become a strange but reassuring ally for Ellen, helping make their lives together feel safe and workable for her despite everything that was changing.

Tim's story reveals a lot about this tricky notion of autonomy. Tim felt that he had the knowledge and ability to decide and control his life. He felt he was able to be autonomous, and that he was acting autonomously. He also expressed how important this was to him, and that he felt that this was a fundamental aspect of how he saw himself. Key parts of this were tied to his driving and his ability to take charge when that was required. These were important aspects of how Tim understood himself within his world. But neither the idea of autonomy nor Tim's story are that simple. There seemed more than a little wisdom in Tim's comment about people not always being the best judge of their capacities. Tim's driving was an important self-expression, but it wasn't clear how he felt about the limits and conditions that he'd agreed and committed to in order to support this. The value he placed on stepping up to "take charge" also seemed difficult to reconcile with how badly it had gone when he'd needed to do this. It was also very clear from Tim's story that Tim wasn't an island or a citadel (images that have often been used to describe how people make decisions and live independently). Tim's story was really Tim and Ellen's story, and considering one without the other wasn't seeing the full picture. Ellen's contributions to their story start to help us to understand how complicated the idea of autonomy can be, particularly when you start to factor in something like dementia. While Tim felt a sense of his capacity and control, there were extra levels to this that he didn't seem to be aware of. Ellen felt that Tim's choices and responses were, due to his faltering memory, actually dictated by her. For Ellen, this wasn't manipulation for her sake but a necessary act for both of them to live well. Many of Tim's choices and responses were not just made by him but came about because of what Ellen was doing, or perhaps not doing through the soft power she had over him in partnership with his memory loss. Ellen's input was also empowering though, as Tim also relied on her in innumerable ways to live his life the way he wanted to. Tim's valued capacity and ability to control his world was solid and compelling while simultaneously being fragile and liable to dissipate, like dense clouds that slowly drift apart leaving nothing to see.

This story reveals quite a lot about autonomy. Autonomy is important and, perhaps because it is so important, it is complicated. It's something that feels important to people and which, for some, might seem central to who they are because of what their choices say about them. But autonomy is easier to describe in theory than in the messiness of our real lives. There is so much that contributes to what choices are made, and reconciling this with a concept of autonomy can be really difficult, particularly when a person has dementia. Nevertheless, the idea of autonomy seems very central to how challenging and worrying dementia is for our community. So now we'll try to explore the ideas behind autonomy a little further to understand why this is the case.

Autonomy — a user's guide to history

The first thing to know when trying to understand autonomy is that, like all complicated ideas, we've been tinkering with it for a long time. Key strides towards how we understand autonomy today were made during the Enlightenment in Europe.[2] Autonomy, at this stage, started to change from something that had been associated traditionally with religious choices and beliefs into something new. This new idea of autonomy was tied up with an increasing fascination with what we know as logic, rationality and scientific ways of knowing. These were key aspects of the then burgeoning concept of truth that had a considerable impact on morality, politics, knowledge and society. Continental European thinkers contributing to this new notion of autonomy (like Voltaire in France, for example) were inspired by what was seen as English progress toward religious tolerance, constitutional government and exciting scientific progress (Popper, 1962). Europe was reeling from the long and destructive impact of the Thirty Years' War and there was an appetite for change and religious, social, and political reform. People started to wonder whether countries and individuals could choose and question their beliefs, rather than just adhering to them. Simultaneously, the scientific method provided new and successful ways to explain the world, making rational thinking seem even more powerful and important than ever before. In this transition, philosophy and natural science changed from being considered as adjuncts to theology to becoming forces that could "challenge the old and construct the new" (Bristow, 2010). Science and objective, rational thinking were becoming regarded optimistically as forces and principles which could solve many of the great human problems and give rise to universally applicable ethics and law (Habermas, 1981). A new kind of valuing developed — a rational humanism — that increasingly considered human interests and reason (coming to an answer through logic and reflection) as central concerns, and that favoured individual autonomy as a key expression of the modern citizen. Within all of this tumult and energy, a concept of personal autonomy arose focused on key notions of agency (free action), rationalism (knowledge arising from reason), and liberty (free choice), ultimately resulting in a view of individuals as "unified, coherent and rational" and authors of their own experience and meaning (Burr, 1995).

A cornerstone for the development of modern autonomy was the work of the German philosopher, Immanuel Kant. This influential foundation also provides a first insight into where some of the difficulties in applying this notion to people with dementia began. Interestingly, different from a lot of later ideas, Kant's autonomy isn't really about freedom but, rather, commitment to rationality. Kant felt that people are duty-bound towards a moral code that is determined by our rational nature (Kant, 1780). Humans might be plagued by irrational impulses, but Kant felt that we can use reason to understand what's best (for us and for people in general) and to support us to follow our own advice. So, the right thing to do is also the thing that we'd rationally decide to do, which is also the thing that we will commit to doing if we are being rational. Kant therefore viewed rationality and autonomy as closely bound together — being autonomous implied being rational and vice versa. From Kant's perspective, how to achieve all of this was to have personal rules that supported universal moral requirements (what would always be good or right). Kant felt that if we could think of a moral rule which was always true and should apply to everyone, following that rule would be the right thing to do.[3] In other words, good autonomy requires our personal rules (e.g. I won't kill people, or I will pay my taxes) to be rational in that it would be a good idea if everyone followed these rules all of the time, and for us to stick to our rules (Kant et al., 2002). Kant's work sowed influential seeds, as links between ideas of rationality and autonomy persist to this day. To have autonomy in Kant's sense, I have to engage with and communicate fairly complicated reasoning about why I'm making a certain choice. We can already see the problems this might create for a person with dementia. This sophisticated and reflective view of rational autonomy hints at the risk that people who are not able to be rational or perhaps, even more worryingly, are at risk of being assumed to be irrational (like people with dementia), won't be seen as autonomous.

What does autonomy mean now?

Kant's association of a moral autonomy with rationality is an important bedrock for how autonomy's meaning has developed, and the challenges this idea has for people with dementia. However, over the years since Kant's time, a vast amount of work and thought has been committed to exploring autonomy and trying to define what it might mean. This has resulted in many different descriptions of autonomy focused on a variety of priorities. A key development from Kant's moral autonomy is that, while his work focused on defining autonomy around whether decisions were right or wrong, or good or bad, a lot of decisions and actions aren't definitely "moral" in that way. More recent work on autonomy has often focused on getting to grips with how and why people do what they do, regardless of whether they're behaving morally. Contemporary descriptions of autonomy often also acknowledge that there might be a difference between an "ideal" sense of autonomy, which might be something we aspire to and work towards possessing, compared with a more universal or basic notion of autonomy that many people possess without needing to work on it. As we discussed earlier, the idea of autonomy has more aspects to it than Kant considered in his work and, even with this richer notion of autonomy, it remains difficult to fit this to real life situations.[4]

• • •

So, why bother talking about all of this? That's a valid question. Primarily it is because the idea of autonomy is incredibly pervasive and powerful and knowing more about it helps make sense of all that dementia means to us. Autonomy, however, is a complicated topic: it can seem overly theoretical, jargonistic and somewhat irrelevant. I've done my best to try to make the following sections relevant and readable, but if you want to take my word for it that our struggles with dementia are made worse by how we think about autonomy, you may wish to skip ahead, and I'll see you at Chapter 4, "Simple principles for a complex space". For those intrepid explorers of autonomy who remain undaunted by warnings of "potentially dry text ahead", I thank you for your company.

Our historically more recent, nuanced ideas of autonomy have implications for people. If you're considered an autonomous person, you're liable to be treated differently and have different laws, statuses and assumptions extended to you than to those deemed not autonomous. Autonomy matters, and therefore the challenges this idea implies for dementia are incredibly important.

If it isn't already clear, autonomy today isn't one single thing that has been agreed upon. There are many different ideas. Some have a lot of overlap and coherence and others less so. Even trying to canvass the variations out there is beyond what we can achieve in this section. So, instead, we're going to try and explore some aspects of how autonomy is considered today from the perspective of two primary ideas. The first is the notion of self-rule, which relates to our ability to make our own choices and then follow them. The second is the notion of independence, which entails our ability to choose or act without being influenced in some way.

Self-rule: when are our decisions and actions our own?

A number of things may be required for our decisions to be regarded as our own. It has been argued that some sort of decision-making competence (which could include our capacity for rational thought, self-control and freedom from things that hamper these — such as a debilitating pathology like dementia) — and authenticity (a kind of reflective coherence of our views, actions and interests) (Christman, 2020) are required. That autonomy should be defined by cognitive competence (that my decisions are thought through or make sense) is central to many ways that questions of autonomy are resolved in law and decision-making processes. It's also worth noting that more recent neuroscientifically-informed views of autonomy have raised questions about how definitively rational and unemotional any person's deliberations in decision-making truly are, thus making the relevance of these traits to personal autonomy uncertain (Felson & Reiner, 2011). Advancing science may change our understanding of this further, but questions of decision-making competence clearly have important implications for dementia, and they interface with the practical question of what we do about all of this in day-to-day life when there are worries about decision-making. We're going to discuss this problem in detail later in Part One.

The other notion of authenticity in autonomy (that my decisions are mine because they align with what's important to me) is interesting and important because it has been influential in how autonomy has been described over the last five decades. For instance, the "hierarchical" views of personal autonomy developed by Harry Frankfurt, Gerald Dworkin, and Wright Neely in the 1970s (J. S. Taylor, 2005a) relied on the fairly simple idea that I'm autonomous when I'm following a reinforcing process where my wishes or desires move me to act. For example, my wish to play the piano (termed a first order desire) is autonomous if it's supported by a second or higher order desire (I want to want to play the piano). In Frankfurt's language, a first order desire that moves me towards an action represents my "will". So, it is my will to play the piano if my desire to do so results in my doing this. From this model Frankfurt defines an autonomous person as one who is capable of these reflective higher-order desires, while a non-person (a "wanton") merely acts on their more spontaneous and less reflective lower-order desires (Frankfurt, 1971).

This simple model seems to have a lot going for it. It enables people to change their preferences for doing things and still be considered autonomous, it doesn't require any rules or powers beyond the individual to describe autonomy, and it allows people to autonomously make decisions which might be considered "bad" choices (on this front a significant departure from Kant) (J. S. Taylor, 2005b). Many technical concerns have been raised regarding this approach: for instance, questions about how we know that a higher order desire is authentic, and how we reconcile multiple conflicting desires (Christman, 1989). It's also been asked what this means if someone was being manipulated (as they were in *The Matrix*) but felt that their choices were authentic (McKenna & Coates, 2015; G. Dworkin, 1976; J. S. Taylor, 2005a). Regardless, this approach to authenticity in autonomy as related to a hierarchy of desires is common and influential.

A different approach to describing authenticity in autonomy is Ekstrom's "coherence theory" (Ekstrom, 1993). Ekstrom's view is that autonomy is not just about how decisions are made, but also how these decisions relate to how we see our "self". Ekstrom felt that our "self" has levels. Our "true self" is an authentic aspect of ourselves where our beliefs and preferences are coherent. Ekstrom suggests that autonomous action occurs when there is coherence between our everyday wishes regarding what we want to do and the preferences of our true self. When these factors cohere, this makes our actions autonomous and also makes those actions self-defining or self-reinforcing. In other words, when what we choose lines up with who we reflectively view ourselves as truly being, we are autonomous.

While relatively simple and intuitively attractive, the various ideas of autonomy as authenticity, when it comes to dementia, can raise some issues for us. What does it mean when cognitive and communicative changes impede detecting or interpreting whether a person's choices are authentic and coherent? Ronald Dworkin has suggested a practical response which highlights a key problem. He felt that earlier choices and preferences should outweigh later ones as dementia progresses, since prior choices will be more informed by the important critical interests of a person. Dworkin viewed dementia as a progression towards being "ignorant of self" and that people with dementia "cannot have projects or plans that leading a critical life requires. They therefore have no contemporary opinion about their own critical interests" (R. Dworkin, 1993: 230). He argued that the cognitive and communicative decline of dementia is inconsistent with autonomy. This has multiple implications. Firstly, this means that we should grant the person with dementia's historic views and preferences the most authority as these reflect the critical interests of the person. Additionally, this paves the way for us to feel justified in disregarding the preferences of people with dementia over time because we would assume that these aren't authentic representations of the person themselves. As we will discuss further, this notion of authenticity has been highly influential and has informed our ethical and legal approaches to people with dementia, but it also creates a number of problems. It sets a high bar for people with dementia as it suggests that, for their preferences and choices to be authentic "critical interests", they must seem understandable and rational to others. In essence, meaning that the person with dementia is responsible for both reflectively generating critical interests and being able to defend these as reasonable to those around them, to be able to be considered autonomous. It also sets up an expectation that a change in preferences for a person with dementia cannot be autonomous. By diminishing the assumed authenticity of choices in advanced dementia we're valuing the past preferences of a person over what they're experiencing and may be expressing right now.

Despite the impact of this approach to considering authenticity and autonomy in dementia, there are powerful alternative views. These can suggest we should refrain from assuming people with dementia don't have interests and authenticity and that we should step back from a cognitively-associated interpretation of autonomy in dementia. It has been suggested that we should be more attuned to the values of people with dementia as central to their autonomy (Jaworska, 1999). Citing the example of a person who wanted to be a research subject owing to a fundamental wish to help others, Jaworska notes that people with dementia can display important personal values. In this way, valuing does not inherently require a static consistency of views over our lives or a strong narrative sense of what we've valued in the past. From this perspective, we can value even if we've lost other cognitive abilities. We should therefore be cautious in assuming that the expressed views of people with dementia are not authentic and not autonomous.

When are we too influenced to be autonomous?

Many people have used the metaphor of the "inner citadel" for autonomy, suggesting a stolid, central and bounded structure. While there may be something intuitively attractive about our own independent and immutable autonomy fortress it's not hard to think of situations that don't fit this metaphor. Decisions and even values seem more fluid and under the influence of many factors than this image seems to imply. A key question then is, what does it mean to have autonomy when we feel or act differently in different situations or at different times. If I have a strong, sustained desire, say, to work in an office after seeing the TV series, *The Office* (2005-13), and an inconsistent equally strong, sustained desire at a different point, say, not to work in an office after seeing *Severance* (2022), are both, either or neither of these wishes autonomous? How much influence is too much for our decisions to be autonomous, and when should we be suspicious if our preferences change?

The American philosopher, Harry Frankfurt, felt that the alignment of what we want to do, our actions and our view of who we are defines an authentic "real self". It is this authentic alignment with who we are now, and not the consistency of the decisions themselves that make them true and autonomous (Wolf, 1993; Frankfurt, 1971). Frankfurt goes further, suggesting that it doesn't necessarily matter if I change my views and actions under the influence of some other factor. A more useful example than the influence of modern television might be Frankfurt's depiction of the "willing addict", a person who was addicted to a drug but was content with their addiction. Despite not being truly "free" to choose, Frankfurt felt that this person remained autonomous despite the influence of addiction as they endorsed their addiction, they wanted to remain addicted, and thus there was still this authentic coherent "mesh" of their closely held wishes and will. This suggests that desires that have been reflected on and reinforced over time can be important and autonomous even if the decisions resulting from them are highly influenced (Christman, 1989; Young, 1986). From this perspective, a decision or an action which is strongly influenced by someone or something outside the person isn't automatically less important since, if the person authentically agrees with what they're being influenced to do, it is still an autonomous act.

Thinking through how much of life is lived without any outside influence seems to heighten the necessity of deciding where autonomy fits into the picture. While Frankfurt's description of a willing drug addict may not be an experience we all relate to, more covert addictions, to social media for example, may feel closer to home. In fact, we're likely more influenced than many of us would be comfortable with. Our increasing understanding of neuroscience indicates that many different influences (either internal or external to the person) radically affect decision-making, raising doubts about whether the "independent", rational ideal has ever been realistic (Felson & Reiner, 2011). Some may argue that the clear influences of culture, family or language, for example, are not undue influences, just parts of who we are and therefore not a risk to an idea like our independent autonomy. Even if we accept that, there are however multiple, subtle influences which routinely and measurably affect what we value and what we decide. For instance, our decisions are often influenced by unconscious, symbolic cues (sometimes referred to as "priming" or "framing") or biases (sometimes referred to as "anchoring") within language or communication (Dubljevic, 2013; Felson & Reiner, 2011). Framing, for instance, occurs when the way the pros and cons of options are "framed" influences the decisions that are made. A healthcare version of this is that people are much more likely to choose a potential medical treatment when they're told 90% of people receiving it are expected to live than if they're told 10% of people are expected to die after receiving it (Armstrong et al., 2002; Felson & Reiner, 2011). We know that messages influence our decisions (would advertising exist if that wasn't true) so where is the threshold at which we lose our autonomy?

At this point our autonomy citadel is starting to look less solid and bounded, seemingly surrounded by, interacting with and composed of a rambling and jumbled town of different structures with varying degrees of permanence. Some newer approaches to autonomy are correspondingly less concerned with the independent rationality of decisions and actions. For instance, in Dubljevic's "post-metaphysical" description of autonomy, the chief concern is the degree of influence and how justifiable the influence is, rather than just that decisions and actions *are* influenced (Dubljevic, 2013). Dubljevic suggests that it would, for instance, be autonomous to act according to society's laws despite their coercive nature. Likewise, compulsions (internal influences) which direct behaviour may not mean a loss of autonomy even if the person is, on occasion, unable to control this impulse (Dubljevic, 2013).

It's important, and reassuring, that we might be able to be autonomous even if we're often more influenced and less rational than we'd like to think. This has implications for everyone, but the implications are even more stark for people with dementia where their autonomy is frequently challenged. People with dementia are often influenced by coercive care, such as in a locked, aged care facility where freedom of movement or activity is limited. This care influences many, but not all, of the choices available to a person with dementia, clearly impacting the ways they can be autonomous. However, if we accept that autonomy and influence can co-exist, a door is opened to describing how people with dementia can remain autonomous in aged care, rather than our having to assume that this is impossible. The idea that people might also remain autonomous despite internal, un-chosen influences ("compulsions" for Dubljevic) is also relevant in dementia. While Dubljevic explores compulsions in relation to a type of dementia (behavioural variant fronto-temporal dementia) his ideas are helpful more generally.[5] He describes levels of compulsion in dementia, such as a mild level which includes the lure of gratification or response to environmental cues — absentmindedly eating conveniently located sweets, or playing with a "fiddle board" (collections of fixed locks, bolts, ties and other familiar objects that some people with dementia like to use), for example. A severe compulsion might be seen when a person with dementia responds to a longer-term deprivation (such as through sexualised behaviour) or past trauma (such as through aggression triggered by physical care acts). Dubljevic also notes that we are all subject to total compulsions where complete physical need (such as the need to be hydrated) influences deeply what we do. Overall, Dubljevic suggests that any adult (including those with dementia) can be both influenced and autonomous and responsible. He recommends that autonomy should only be in question if we are confident that the influence is one that the person and others couldn't agree with and validly include within their longer-term plan for themselves, if they had the chance to reflect on it (Dubljevic, 2020).

Reflecting on this problem invites us to wonder how an internal influence ("compulsion") could be consistent with a long-term life-plan of a person with dementia and not diminish their autonomy. I think my experiences with Patrick, a man in his 70s with advanced dementia who lived in an aged care facility, provide an example.

Patrick had been a medical doctor earlier in his life but had discovered a love of art and painting in his later years after he had been diagnosed with dementia. His art was beautiful. He painted pictures of his beloved garden and made frames by hand out of bits of native timber. One picture seemed like a portrait. A single figure alone sat in an armchair in a sitting room. I couldn't tell whether the figure was meant to be Patrick or someone else, but I always thought of that picture when I visited him. The hunched, pale figure in the painting surrounded by Patrick's paintings of his garden seemed to have some oracular power, a foreshadowing of a future Patrick sitting alone at a table next to a window in an aged care facility.

Whenever I visited Patrick at the facility he was usually sitting at that same table. Agapanthus crowded the space outside and pressed up against the glass so much that, from one angle, he appeared to be sitting within their lush tapering leaves. Patrick could walk when he wanted to, but he usually seemed content to sit at his sunny garden table. Patrick could no longer speak. His dementia had diminished his language, causing him to lose words and ideas until it seemed he had nothing he wanted to try to say. But Patrick wasn't *just* sitting there. At his table Patrick was actively doing. And, while he couldn't speak, it didn't mean he had nothing to try and communicate. Patrick was creating. He would arrange objects on the table in front of him. Pens, cutlery, books, whatever was available. He would take the objects he had and place them down in front of him on the table. He'd look at what was there and then he'd adjust them this way, then that, and then another way, pausing each time and considering his work between constructing each new variation. Each new item extended the complexity of his creation, being added into the repertoire of its form. But whatever the meaning of this activity may have been for Patrick, it was not static. The work required constant consideration and adjustment responsive to qualities and considerations that were intangible to others, and otherwise inexpressible for Patrick.

Patrick could not explain what he was doing. Due to his advanced dementia, he wasn't able to speak or write to tell us what doing this meant for him, nor what he felt it should mean for us. Patrick's arrangements seem consistent with Dubljevic's notion of a mild compulsion in that he was (from our perspective) spontaneously engaging with his environment. However, these actions were also considered, purposeful and coherent with Patrick's pre-existing life-plan, relating to his interest in self-expression through art. While Patrick may have been in no doubt about the purpose of his art for him, a challenge in dementia (that we've discussed) is that autonomy and the value of experiences for people with dementia tend to be determined by others, not the person themselves. Interpreting these moments of construction as "art" relied not just on his having an audience but that audience knowing enough about Patrick to know that these actions could be fragile gestures towards his prevailing wishes and values (Chapman et al., 2019). We can see, and Dubljevic argues, that the presence of compulsions may affect autonomy in dementia, but not all compulsions and not all of the time. Additionally, autonomy may not always be about individuals but can be a result of how we are together.

Relational autonomy

This idea, that autonomy relies to some degree on the mesh of human relationships rather than is somehow separate from them, is a newer way to think about autonomy. This "relational" view accepts autonomy as something that exists within the intermeshed cultural and social experiences lived by us all (Mackenzie & Stoljar, 2000). Relational autonomy is also often seen as a critical response to earlier "fundamentally individualistic and rationalistic" or "standard" views of autonomy (such as those we've explored from Frankfurt and Dworkin) which are seen as reliant on a "mythic" illusion of the independence of individuals (Nedelsky, 2011; Gomez-Virseda et al., 2019).

Relational views of autonomy, which have been developed by feminist thinkers, explicitly focus on the barriers to autonomy that arise through oppression, both from internal and external or social sources (Stoljar, 2013). Autonomy from this perspective arises as a factor of the relationships that we have with those around us, our culture and our society (Gomez-Virseda et al., 2019). This approach does not remove the individual from the centre of consideration but sees our environment of personal relationships as the ground that enables — or hinders — our developing the skills and capacities through which we achieve the status of being self-determining and responsible (Donchin, 2000).

It will come as no surprise to anyone who has made it this far along the journey through this chapter that even a subset of approaches to autonomy, in this case relational autonomy, is complicated and there are multiple views and perspectives. American philosopher Friedman's relational approach sees relationships as central to autonomy.

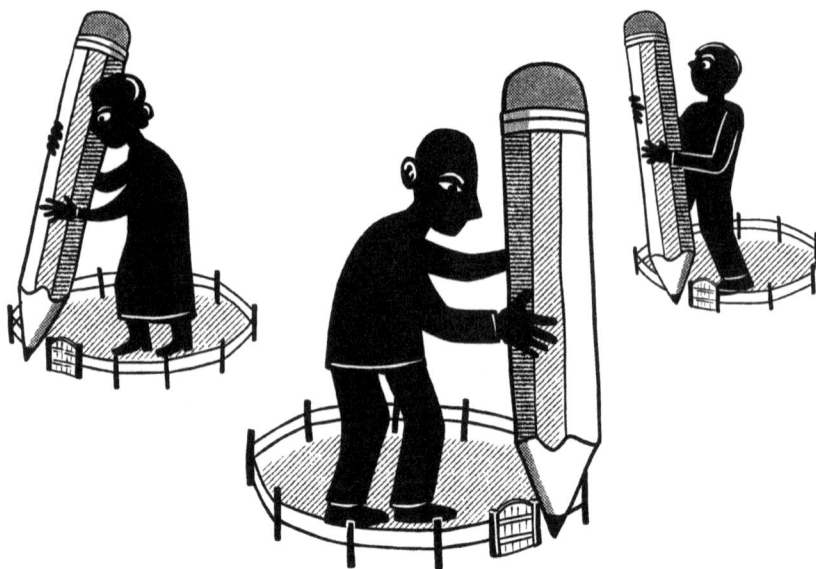

Relationships with friends and family can enhance or diminish an individual's capacity for autonomy. Relationships also impact upon whether our choices can be seen as "good" moral choices — which has implications for whether we should be considered autonomous (Stoljar, 2013). Our relationships and how we conduct them are central to how we comport ourselves (M. Oshana, 2006). Autonomy might also be something that results from how we are brought up, and the circumstances that surround us, and not just from processes that we control (Baier, 1985). From this perspective our social experiences influence when autonomy can be present and whether autonomy is even possible. Being a slave might mean we can never direct ourselves or have the context required to be considered autonomous (M. A. L. Oshana, 1998; Brison, 2000). Autonomy, considered in this relational way, raises a different set of questions for people with dementia. A diminished focus on independence and rationality along with tolerance of the notion of influence seems to make it easier to argue that a relational notion of autonomy could indeed persist in dementia. Dementia has a considerable impact on relationships (as we shall see) but the potential for relationships to adapt and be supported hints at important possibilities in responding to dementia.

Autonomy: a safe and settled concept?

Several things should now be clear: that autonomy is something we value, that humanity has been working on this problem for a while, and that we haven't been able to simplify it into one idea. We don't have a single and accepted way of describing autonomy and who has it. More critically, we don't have a perfect way of describing or knowing how to make universal sense of autonomy. We might be confident that we — the readers of these pages — are autonomous, but what about all of those other people who seem different? How do we know if they have autonomy? Deciding is risky. Autonomy tends to be an idea that's worked on and thought about by highly educated and privileged people, but it has the greatest implications for those with the greatest disadvantages. Those most at risk from ways of interpreting autonomy have likely always been the disadvantaged, and (as we shall see for people with dementia) that challenge remains. The stakes are high and a simple and perfect explanation for autonomy probably isn't just around the corner.

However, while there are a lot of different approaches to autonomy, as we've described, there's also coherence amongst them. The overlapping nature of many newer models of autonomy demonstrates that we are "on the right track" to describing it in a way which will be broadly accepted (J. S. Taylor, 2005a). Certainly, many contemporary descriptions of autonomy have a more nuanced idea of the role of influence and tend to focus on the person's own reflective involvement in their own decisions and actions as being central to determining autonomy. It's more debatable whether these ideas have permeated our collective understanding of autonomy and affected our views as deeply as the more individualistic and rational notion of autonomy. Regardless, this developing sense that a key element of autonomy lies within our ability to reflect on and respond to our experience is important and may lead to significant changes. The work of Cornelius Castoriadis (a French-Greek philosopher, social critic, economist and psychoanalyst) suggests that autonomy lies within self-reflective processes where people and societies develop through responding to challenges. For Castoriadis, autonomy is not specifically related to the choices made by an individual or a society but through a whole "project" of reflective development (Castoriadis, 1991: 163).

The notion of autonomy as a reflective project appealingly suggests that we should be considering autonomy as continuum and as a work in progress rather than something that is determined as either present or absent at a particular point (Gomez-Virseda et al., 2019). It also seems to open space for autonomy to be considered as something beyond the activity of a "solitary citadel". Autonomy may be under the influence of people other than the person being scrutinised and still be present and be valuable. Although it is an odd thing to say at the end of a long chapter devoted to the importance of autonomy, it's not the only important thing about being a person. There are many other values and qualities which are critical to how we are and how we see each other — such as compassion, hope, trust, empathy, solidarity and responsibility (Gomez-Virseda et al., 2019). We might all agree that these qualities and values are important. They may not be as powerful and influential, however, as autonomy has been in determining what statuses we extend to each other.

The tyranny of norms: valuing people

Whether we think a person has autonomy matters for many reasons. However, the most critical reason for us here is that whether we believe a person has autonomy or not affects how we treat and value them. This is where our thinking about autonomy (what we understand of the idea of self-governance and what that means to us) starts to take on a more focused ethical component which, in this case, includes questions like, what value do we place on autonomy in a person and is that the right value and the right approach to valuing a person.[6]

During the time of the Ancient Greeks, personal autonomy was valued when it reflected and reinforced society's notion of how to live well (Ashley, 2012). This ancient type of autonomy related to belonging and cohesively contributing to a community. By comparison, many contemporary (particularly "individualistic") approaches to valuing autonomy seem to focus on liberty — living by our own terms — as key to determining its worth. It seems that if I act to express my autonomy (through a focus on my individual needs and wants) I seem to elevate my worth and my value. The shift here, from valuing actions and desires which cohere with and relate to others, to valuing actions and desires in a way that is regardless of others is critical. Today, living by your own "free" standards is highly valued, potentially regardless of the impact on others, and potentially regardless of its impact on your own safety and community protection.[7] Importantly, however, individualistic autonomy is not only commonly considered valuable, it is also considered normal. By this reckoning, I'm a normal person with a good life if I live it on my individualistic terms and if we believe that our society should value that experience.

This line of thinking raises important questions: who are the normal, "autonomous", valuable people and who are not and in what ways are they more or less valuable? Discussions within the bioethics literature on these points highlight some immediate problems that seem to be associated with conflating autonomy and normality. Non-autonomous people within bioethics discussions frequently include infants and children, people in a coma, people with major cognitive impairment or mental illness, and people with drug addictions. All of us will fit into at least one of those camps at some point, and many of us will have experienced periods of time in multiple of them. Am I only normal and valuable now because I'm a middle-aged man with no major illnesses or addictions that our society is worried about? (If coffee has made the list by the time you're reading this, then I might not scrape in.)

Interestingly, being an employed professional with an income also probably doesn't hurt in my attempt at being "normal". Not being a current member of an "ab-normal" group isn't all there is to say about being normal. While we might all hope to be normal, some of us are more normal than others. Modern individualistic ideas are often combined with a cultural focus on consumerism and perpetual growth as a demonstration of "success" and good living. Many lives don't fit the bill. [8] We're normal not just because we make self-determined choices but by expressing those choices through the things we buy and consume, and the wealth we possess. The challenge for the "normality" of older people, who may be more reliant on others and who may no longer have the income they used to have is obvious. Not only do many modern societies tend to diminish the value of people as they age, we also now suggest they aspire to a consumerist "postmodern timelessness" where "successful" ageing means a person doesn't change, but remains vital, powerful and engaged (Katz & Marshall, 2003). In the film *Las Vegas*, four ageing actors (Kevin Cline, Michael Douglas, Robert De Niro, and Morgan Freeman) play four ageing men seeking to reconnect and celebrate the upcoming marriage of one of their number to a much younger woman (Turteltaub, 2013). They party, attempt to seduce other younger women and spend money in glitzy Las Vegas with the story interspersed by comic references to their ageing.

While superficially celebrating the notion of "successful ageing", this film actually highlights an alternative message (Scheidt, 2015.). With its preview banner line of "It's never too late for the party of a lifetime" this film reminds us that the ageing we value is an ageing that resists ageing or being old. This fantastic view glosses over the realities and challenges of ageing while additionally highlighting two populations of older people that require different treatment, those who are self-actualised and worthy of support and a dependent population who are of less worth, while ironically requiring more support (Rubinstein & De Medeiros, 2015). In our consumer-focused contemporary society, being independent means being economically productive, and those who are best able to fulfil these roles are affirmed and rewarded (Post, 2006). This adds an extra level of disadvantage and challenge when we're considering people with dementia who are likely to be considered as worth less than others because of their cognitive impairment and likely dependence, but also because they're also unlikely to be demonstrating the independence we value through living a consumerist lifestyle.

Autonomy and normality are therefore ideas which align with certain privileges (Frey, 2005). A normal, autonomous individual is considered a "citizen" and has worth and rights. Martha Nussbaum, a philosopher whose work we will explore further soon, argues that the idea of independent autonomy is a powerful "fiction" which leads us to valuing some people over others. It influences what we consider as just and fair even though it's just a story we tell each other (Nussbaum, 2004: 310). Contributing to this story are ideas about how members of a society should work together. The philosopher, John Locke, for instance, felt that a good society works by social contracts or mutual obligations between people and the state where participants are "free, equal and independent" (Locke, 1764). This focus makes it seem a little unclear how or if we need to include within our obligations to each other people whom we don't consider free, equal or independent. John Rawls, another philosopher influential in contemporary thinking about how societies should work, felt that societies should be fair, and that equal justice should be available to every moral person. He suggests that everyone who could or does have the capability for a sense of justice and a conception of their personal good through a rational life plan should be considered a moral person who deserves justice, clearly intending his notion of justice to be broadly inclusive (Rawls, 2006). But Rawls also saw citizens as "fully cooperating members of a society over a complete life", which further challenges what sort of status and value we should extend to the many who are unable to continue to cooperate "normally" (Rawls, 2005: 20). The powerful story of individual autonomy is a central contributor to whom we decide is normal enough to deserve justice, be a citizen and be considered worthwhile and valuable. This story raises the stakes for more vulnerable members of society whose autonomy may be questioned (Nussbaum, 2009).

So, what can we say about autonomy after this discussion? It is valuable to our societies and within our societies to be an autonomous person. However, our ideas about who these attributes and statuses should apply to and why are far less clear. There's also an important tradition of thinking about autonomy which associates it with characteristics (like being rational) which make it difficult for many people (like people with dementia) to be considered as autonomous by others. These descriptions and statuses, largely bestowed by one person or one society on another person or people, have significant implications for how we understand and treat each other. This is true for all people ("normal" or otherwise), but the stakes are even higher for people with physical, cognitive and social vulnerabilities, characteristics all of which may be possessed by people with dementia. What we haven't discussed explicitly, although it may be very obvious to you already, is that the loudest voices within discussions about autonomy and normality (indeed all of the experts that we've referred to thus far) would be assuming that they were autonomous, they were normal. That's certainly true for me writing this book and, I'd assume, probably true of you who are reading it. Ideas about autonomy and normality are usually stories that we're telling about someone else, someone whom we feel is different and whom we feel we may need to treat differently because of this. This is a subtle and important point for reflection that we'll continue to explore, but perhaps we can start to see some extra problems that emerge with that thought. If it is the "normal" autonomous people making rules for others with more risks and disadvantages, couldn't that lead to extra problems, and greater risks?

4. Simple decisions for a complex space

Many of the ideas which we have explored together thus far have related to ethics (or moral philosophy), in itself a huge topic but often thought of as involving the way we think and talk about, justify and govern the things that we do.

Ethics, like any area of human endeavour, isn't a fixed and static thing. Much has changed over time. This is true of all categories of ethics, but very true of applied ethics which is the category of ethics that focuses on figuring out what's best to do in particular situations. There are a number of different types of applied ethics but the one that we're most interested in for this discussion is bioethics. Bioethics is a surprisingly recent term. There are numerous different definitions, but you could think of bioethics as the study of what we should do, think and say relating to the biological issues and facts concerning people and animals. Much of the discussion of ethics and philosophy that we've engaged in so far has really been about how to think about big, somewhat general, questions and problems, like what does autonomy mean and what does it involve. As an applied ethics, bioethics is more involved in the next question: "what does that mean for this person or this situation?" For instance, now that we have an idea of what autonomy might mean or might encompass, what does that mean for how we care for other people? While a relative newcomer to the field of moral philosophy, bioethics has had its own part to play in influencing how we think about those whom we have considered autonomous or not, and about dementia in particular — and what we do.

Ethics has always been part of caring for people, and people have been involved in providing healthcare of some sort to themselves and each other for millennia. So, from that perspective we've always been engaging with bioethics in trying to sort out the "what to do" questions that are part of providing care. However, bioethics as a discrete term and area of focused study has had quite a short history. Bioethics arose from an increased focus on social equality and medical and institutional transparency within a particular social and cultural context. In the US, a centre for the development of modern bioethics, this was catalysed by the experiences of the Nuremberg Trials;[9] multiple failures in research and institutional ethical practises; and a need to develop approaches to challenges arising from new technologies (like the invention of kidney dialysis) (Beecher, 1966).[10]

From this background, a specific form of bioethics gained prominence. This form of bioethics, principlism, was developed by Tom Beauchamp (a philosopher) and James Childress (an ethicist). It included four pillars that govern ethical conduct: respect for autonomy, beneficence, non-maleficence, and justice (Beauchamp & Childress, 1994). Refreshingly, after our long and complex discussion of autonomy in the previous chapter, within principlism autonomy has been described more briefly as being present when a person is free from constraint and when they possess a capacity for choice. This far simpler notion of autonomy was subsequently clarified by Beauchamp. To consider a person's action as autonomous from his perspective, three conditions need to be present, namely, that the action is intentional, understood and voluntarily undertaken (Beauchamp, 2005). Unsurprisingly, principlist bioethics also suggests that autonomous decisions and actions have value, and these types of decisions should be respected.

Principlism and autonomy

Principlist bioethics is a huge success story. It is incredibly well known and very popular. If someone feels they know something about health ethics it is probably something related to these four principles. It has justifiably been commended for its clarity, simplicity, and its broad applicability (Gillon, 2003b). It is also taught almost universally to healthcare providers, and many people (clinicians and otherwise) consider these four principles as encompassing all of healthcare ethics. Principlism is, however, not without controversy. It has been argued that it is too simple and easy. It is (for some) a shorthand for a collection of ethical theories which lacks a central coherence, neglects significant issues and bypasses practical concerns due to its central focus of aiming to be widely applicable (Clouser & Gert, 1990). Principlism has also been charged with neglecting emotional and personal factors, over-simplifying problems, and excessively assuming its universal applicability (Campbell, 2003).

A central target part of principlism is the principle of respect for autonomy. This has been argued by many as being the most important part of principlism ("the first among equals") (Gillon, 2003a), and certainly it continues to have a significant and complex impact on healthcare. Respect for autonomy makes sense on many levels. People receiving healthcare, as independent decision-makers, should have their decisions respected and should feel confident that they'll be informed adequately to make the best decisions. When we're unable to make decisions for ourselves our wishes should continue to be respected even if others need to be more involved in decision-making. This makes sense, at least in part because principlism has successfully influenced how we think about and work through these kinds of challenges in healthcare. But it is clear that this approach to autonomy includes problematic assumptions, namely, that people are essentially independent and that rationality is the most important and valuable aspect of decision-making. As we saw in the last chapter, those are fairly debatable points, and assuming their truth has implications.

Let's dig into the principle of respecting autonomy in a little more detail. First, how is autonomy defined? Beauchamp has described the version of autonomy he developed with Childress as separate from moral considerations. By this he means that it's best to define autonomy based on whether a person has particular mental or psychological qualities (that is, determining whether their decision is rational) rather than moral aspects (like whether their decisions are good decisions for them or for others) (Beauchamp, 1999). But there are a number of things to respond to here. It's arguable how confident we can be about the mental and psychological qualities required for a decision to be valid (we're going to discuss this in detail next chapter). It's arguable whether this kind of rationalist definition of autonomy is valid (we explored this in detail last chapter). Many versions of autonomy suggest that relational and social experiences, rather than just individual mental ones, are very central to how we should think about this concept. It's also arguable how much we can ever separate assessment of these sorts of cognitive and psychological qualities from some sort of social valuing of the person's decision, or the person themselves. Societies have a rich tradition of assigning moral status and worth (including, as we've seen, the idea of "normality") based on these kinds of qualities. Saying that we can separate assessment of cognitive and psychological qualities from the values that societies assume seems unrealistic. Overall, many have argued that, in the quest for simplicity, the principlist notion of autonomy ignores much that's very important.

In defending against these sorts of concerns, Beauchamp and Childress have stressed that their principles argue that autonomy should be respected rather than trying to claim how we should understand autonomy (Beauchamp & Childress, 1994). That already makes the simplicity of the principle less clear, as it is more challenging to respect something if we're not sure how to identify it. If something is as important as respect for autonomy, then ideally it would be correspondingly clear (Donchin 2001). Without this clarity you'd wonder (as many have) whether the principles could be used in an unintended way to justify the opinions of individual people in response to healthcare decisions rather than achieving (as they've intended to) some sort of more reliable and universal approach to deciding that we can be confident about (Lee, 2010). But let's take on board the point that principlists don't want to define autonomy for us but want us to focus on showing respect for it. Firstly, you may be validly wondering what we mean by showing respect or how easy it is to respect a person's choice or action if it doesn't seem to be consistent with some sort of social norm. Part of the root of their approach here might come from thinkers like John Stewart Mill who felt that autonomy was intrinsically tied to the notion of personal freedom and that these both contribute to well-being and a good life (Mill, 1859). Good living, from this perspective, results from exercising freedom and our collective task is, to some extent, to get out of each other's way and allow freedom to happen. Respect for autonomy, then, could be considered as a claim that we should support the primary importance of freedom in decision-making. This is certainly one of the ways this principle seems to be interpreted in many contexts. Some have suggested that this contributes to a "moral vacuum" where our ability to share values and think and compromise together about human problems is abandoned when we embrace the apparently simple virtue of personal choice in healthcare (McCormick, 1999). It's also been suggested that this promotion of free, individual healthcare decisions arises from a notion that health outcomes are based on individual choices and that healthcare decisions are between free, independent men meeting as doctor and patient. Thus, respect for autonomy risks ignoring all the structural reasons, disadvantages and vulnerabilities which aren't choices but do impact the choices that we have available to us (Azétsop & Rennie, 2010). In effect, this perspective suggests that prioritising a respect for autonomy might miss all the challenges that impair and impact the autonomy of many people (like people with dementia) who aren't the "normal" people envisaged within these individualistic models. This central focus on the importance of free decision-making, while it makes sense to many cultural groups like white Americans, isn't necessarily as important in other cultures and contexts, further challenging how confident we can be that, by approaching the problem in this way, we're doing something that will always be applicable (Chattopadhyay & De Vries, 2008; Donchin, 2001; Lee, 2010).

So, is respect for autonomy a bad idea? No, clearly not. We should remember that bioethics arose from an era of paternalism and poor ethical conduct. A focus on respecting autonomy was an important counterbalance to central concerns of that time. Perhaps then, it's more accurate to say that the way this idea has been developed and disseminated has created many unintended problems. It could certainly be more valuable than it often is at the moment. It would be a lot more useful if we considered respect for autonomy as an ideal that we needed to work hard to achieve, including by accepting a broader understanding of autonomy than the individualistic and rational one that's usual (Donchin, 2001). This would help us avoid the assumptions within principlism which are routinely overlooked when healthcare ethics means "ticking off the principles". However, as is, principlism assumes norms that are not the experience for many. Principlism also seems to invite us to remain uncertain about what sorts of expressions and lived experiences (in those at risk of being determined as "ab-normal") are valid for inclusion, or worse, to not wonder about this at all. In effect, principlism (and its conception of autonomy) inadvertently contributes to systems of meaning and assumptions which can further disadvantage or dis-empower those already at risk of remaining unheard or misunderstood (Sherwin, 1998). Despite principlism's uptake and appeal as a simple way of applying ethical ideas to healthcare situations it's problematic and contains a lot of implications for people with dementia.

What does this mean for the "ab-normal"?

As we've noted, the bioethics of principlism is based on multiple assumptions, primarily that autonomy is related to ideas of freedom and rational thinking, that the status we derive from autonomy is highly valuable, and that these are normal qualities of people. However, as Martha Nussbaum notes, these elements may not be as assured as they seem on face value. She contends that the common concept of the "citizen as a competent, independent adult" may be a myth (Nussbaum, 2004: 311). Nussbaum believes that the societal tensions between the "normal" and "unusual" states of dependence are things that we all contribute to fabricating. There are many reasons why we do this, but a central one is likely to be that we don't like thinking about being dependent or getting sicker or dying. Actually, we're generally terrified by these ideas and spend a good deal of our lives actively avoiding spending any time at all thinking about the fact that this is, quite literally, going to happen to all of us. Appreciating being (relatively) healthy and (somewhat) independent as "normal" allows some cognitive breathing room between how we feel now and those other "unusual" states that we really don't want to think about. That person, our thinking goes, who's a little older than me and is more dependent than me, isn't me. They're different. They're not like the slightly younger "normal" person who doesn't have those problems yet. It all seems a bit thin and desperate when you write it out like that, doesn't it, but we all do it. As Nussbaum notes, we are all amazingly capable of ignoring the fact that our lives are necessarily interdependent with others and that they feature completely reliable and absolutely normal periods of "helplessness". These affect everyone at the extremes of age and many of us at other times. As much as we might not like it, being dependent and being reliant on others is a normal human experience, it's just the degree of this that varies.

The usual individualistic view of autonomy doesn't have a lot of room for this focus. Actually, it contributes to our "illusion of independence", a feat which forms an important part of our evaluation of worth in our society (Harrigan & Gillett, 2009). Further, it has been argued that "normal" is an idea we create — something that is common sense to us but is actually specific to our society (Elliott, 1999). Elliott makes a comparison with the island of Martha's Vineyard in the United States which, historically, had a high number of deaf persons and where, up until the early-mid 20th century, both sign language and English were considered normal communication. You weren't disabled if you were deaf at that time in Martha's Vineyard, you were normal. Based on this example, Elliott suggests that deafness is not a handicap because of the impairment itself, but due to our society's heavy reliance on verbal communication to function "normally". If our society were different, then our sense of normal would substantially shift. If our society were more focused on acknowledging and supporting the normality of dependence, it would be normal to us. But without our conscious attention or intent, our assumptions and biases mutually reinforce themselves, and our feelings that ageing and dependency are abnormal perpetuate that story, making it much harder to hear alternatives.

Dementia doesn't just mean dependence, though. There are other challenges, like changes in thinking and communication which seem harder still to fit into a sense of "normal". It is worth reminding ourselves, however, that not being able to appreciate what an experience is like doesn't mean that there is no experience there. Frey talked about the idea that human lives are valuable in part because they include "rich content", and implied here is that we all contribute to deciding or assuming whether someone else's experience includes this "rich content" (Frey, 2005). Determining what another person's experience includes is difficult, particularly if they can't help you by telling you about it, and if their experiences seem very different to those that you have and value. Previously, we discussed the story of Patrick, the man with dementia and latter year artist who made and changed arrangements of objects on his table. Patrick's arrangements seemed like art to me and, I'd argue, could have been a "rich" experience for him but were equally easily disregarded by many as purposeless and valueless. Not being able to understand another being creates the space for us to fill that silence with our own stories. What those stories include depend largely on our broader values and our choices about how they apply to the current situation. It's common in ethical and philosophical literature focused on autonomy to assume that a person's experience lacks or has diminished meaningful content when communication seems challenging. An example is the inclusion of infants and pre-verbal children in descriptions of non-autonomous, "unusual" states. But these states may also have a richer content than we usually appreciate. There is an increasing understanding that the life of infants before they develop language is rich and complex. Based on detailed studies of infants, rather than on easily observable behaviour, Daniel Stern has suggested that infants' sense of self may develop well prior to any communicative ability to express this to others (Stern, 1998). In making these observations I'm not claiming that all people with advanced dementia have rich inner lives. However, I would note that our usual societal assumptions that people with dementia and other "ab-normal" people who don't seem to have "normal" experiences that we find valuable creates a risk that we may overlook or misunderstand their experiences.

For all the good achieved by bioethics, a focus on principlism as our key model for understanding it has contributed to significant problems. This is primarily due to its reliance on a notion of autonomy intertwined with assumptions of personal rationality and individual independence, neither of which is true for everyone nor always helpful. This has contributed to an environment where those whose needs and experiences don't align with this model, notably, for us, people with dementia, are at risk of being misunderstood or devalued. Examples of this are, unfortunately, readily apparent as we shall see.

5. Decisions and dementia: hearing, learning and supporting

Having laid this groundwork we can now start to hone in upon exactly what our valuing of an individualistic view of autonomy, and the associated implications for bioethics and the kinds of cultural assumptions about what it is to have a "normal" life, means for how we respond to a problem like dementia. In this chapter, we'll explore the implications of these issues for how we think about and support decision-making capacity in dementia, and what we consider intelligible from people with dementia during these processes; we'll assess what decisions mean and express for people with dementia; and we'll analyse what this means for how we undertake research with people with dementia to understand their experience.

Before we begin, however, let's return to Nancy's story.

As the years passed, there seemed to be more people worried for Nancy for more and more reasons. She remained strong and determined in her convictions, but it became clearer over time that things were getting difficult for her. It was clear that Nancy was becoming more dependent on others and her staying at home was getting riskier.

In the words of Kerrie, Nancy's GP, she needed a "constant person", someone dependable who'd be there for her and who would help her to be where she wanted to be. Nancy was surrounded by people, but very few seemed able or keen to step up. Nancy wasn't particularly flexible and didn't want to be helped. She'd also had a lifelong habit of deciding that some things others would consider very important weren't of interest to her and so she'd just ignore them. For instance, as passionate and inspiring as she was as an artist, she was completely disinterested in this being a profession. People wanted to pay her for her work, which she knew was a good thing, but she wasn't interested in keeping track of any of this. Her family "got rid" of many of her works for her, selling them overseas. Nancy didn't lack for money because of this, but the feelings that she'd been taken advantage of started early and the worry only grew as the years passed.

Victoria, Nancy's oldest friend, arose from all of this mess and took a central part in sorting out the bits of Nancy's life that

Nancy wasn't interested in. She started booking shows, organising sales and managing Nancy's money. Eventually, this situation was formalised with Victoria becoming Nancy's manager and legal decision-maker. This worked well for years until Victoria developed her own health problems and felt she couldn't continue. At this point, they were both in their eighties and Nancy's memory and her temper had been deteriorating for some time. Victoria felt incredibly guilty at the thought of letting her friend down and felt she couldn't talk to Nancy about this until she had sorted out a solution. The solution, it turned out, was Rosie.

Rosie met Nancy when she came on as her cleaner. Rosie and her husband had a cleaning business and Rosie had visited the house weekly for many years. Over time, Rosie and Nancy became friends and both looked forward to their weekly time together. Rosie never anticipated that this would result in her becoming a carer and support person for Nancy. This change just seemed to happen, arriving unexpectedly and unavoidably. Victoria knew she couldn't leave Nancy in the lurch, so she asked and eventually begged Rosie to take on this central decision-making role in her friend Nancy's life. Rosie was reluctant and, when Nancy eventually found out, she was furious. However, Rosie decided to help and Nancy came to rely on her and trust her deeply.

The new role was as difficult for Rosie as she had worried it would be. Not so much because of Nancy but because of her wanting to be absolutely clear that she wasn't inadvertently taking advantage of Nancy, and because of Nancy's family's frequent innuendo that she was. While they'd been absent for much of her life her siblings, it seemed to Rosie's and Nancy's eyes, became more interested in her as she became frailer. Rosie was scrupulous in making and documenting every decision and expense with Nancy's close input whenever she could coax that attention.

Rosie didn't want to put a foot out of place, Nancy was fiercely independent, and even Nancy's GP, Kerrie, felt that her medical role should be to wait until something happened, rather than to suggest that a change was required. It seemed as though Nancy would stay in the big, empty old house until a fall or some other catastrophe robbed her of an alternative. But then, the decision that Nancy would leave was made. Everyone felt that they'd been the one who'd made it and all at the same time. Rosie felt she'd supported Nancy to realise that her safety was really at risk, and Kerrie felt that it had been her clearly stating her medical opinion that leaving was the right thing to do that had moved the situation forward. Kerrie now believed that Nancy no longer had the capacity to make a decision to stay, meaning that Rosie now seemed to be reluctantly responsible for the decision (as Nancy's appointed surrogate decision-maker) that Nancy should live in a facility. At the same time, Nancy felt she'd decided that enough was enough. She said, "I made the decision in the end. I realised I just had enough intelligence left to realise that I'd have to be sensible about it". For Nancy this was a response to her childhood feelings of isolation and being pushed around. The decision to move into safety and support now made deep sense to her, even when the alternative had seemed so clearly "right" to her for the many difficult, preceding years.

Nancy's story raises all sorts of questions. Nancy felt that she was acting autonomously. She felt that she had been driving decisions to stay at home and be unsafe, to be supported by people other than her family, and then to move to the facility. In this brief narrative, different interpretations of each of these points are clearly present, including within a legal and clinical framework, which had determined that Nancy no longer had the capacity to make these decisions. And yet, Nancy felt she did have capacity and that what was decided fitted with the life that she felt she had lived. The contradictions and complexities in this story highlight how challenging it is to make sense of what concepts like autonomy and capacity mean in practice, concepts which can seem simultaneously irrelevant and powerfully binding when we are relating to the real lived experience of people with dementia.

Decision-making and capacity in dementia

Principlism's focus on autonomy arose from a need to attend to patients' rights and respond to medical paternalism. From the mid-twentieth century, there was broad legal and philosophical support for considering a focus on autonomy as of key importance. Such theoretical perspectives were taken as evidence that more focus on the independent choices of patients would be welcome and empowering (Peisah et al., 2013). However, the decades since have not seen the desired outcome. Patients may be less, rather than more, empowered as physicians, responding to their interpretation of how to respect independent patient autonomy, have withheld their expert opinions for fear of unduly influencing patients (Kim, 2010). Patients have therefore often been left with difficult decisions to make, but without adequate supports or guidance (Quill & Brody, 1996). It has even been argued that such a focus on "stark autonomy" diminishes patients' autonomy by removing a patient's power to choose not to be involved in choosing anything at all (Loewy, 2005). For all its intent, principlism has not succeeded in empowering patients as had been hoped (Loewy, 2005).

The challenges (and deficiencies) of principlist autonomy are amplified when considering the needs of older persons and those with cognitive impairments like dementia. There has been discussion about the difficulty of fitting the needs of older and more dependent people within the current political and theoretical interpretation of autonomy in healthcare (Agich, 2003). An "interstitial" view of autonomy that views human experience as a multitude of interdependencies occurring all of the time has been suggested as preferable. Autonomy would be more useful for older people if it valued our interdependencies and understood decisions as more than a need for independent response to milestone moments (such as the potential need for a move to an aged care facility to receive additional help) (Agich, 2003).

While an "interstitial" interpretation of autonomy seems a helpful step forward, it is challenging to fit this to current frameworks and the usual responses to common problems. This isn't a criticism of this way of thinking about autonomy, necessarily, but an acknowledgement that most systems are based on different ideas, and fitting an interstitial view of autonomy into these would involve considerable change.

How we decide

As we've discussed (and conscious of the relevance of an interstitial view of autonomy for this population), capacity assessments only help with a discrete set of problems associated with cognitive changes. Usually, approaches to decision-making for people with dementia and those around them change as a natural and somewhat organic response to what's occurring well before any capacity assessment is judged to be needed. Involvement of others in decision-making for a person with dementia tends to increase over time (Hirschman et al., 2004). How persons with dementia are involved and what influence this has upon what is decided is complex, and unpredictable, and it's often difficult to know who made the final decision. Often, all that seems clear is that a decision has been made (Sugarman et al., 2001). But this can be a process that's constructive and even beneficial for all those involved. It's been noted that good collaborative, shared approaches to decision-making can, in effect, increase a person with dementia's autonomy by increasing their engagement with the decision-making process (Whitlatch & Menne, 2009). Approaching decisions relationally, that is working them through together, can have multiple potential benefits for a person with dementia and their care networks, including greater rating of well-being, quality of life, lower levels of depression and less strain on caregivers (Whitlatch & Menne, 2009; Menne et al., 2008; Menne et al., 2002). How this works best within networks of people with dementia and those around them is understandably affected by a number of factors such as quality of relationships, decision-making style and the value placed on individual autonomy (High, 1992).

While these processes often work, that doesn't mean that they are always easy for those involved. Families and carers can often feel under-supported or under-involved in decision-making particularly in relation to healthcare choices (Gessert et al., 2000; Givens et al., 2009). The burden of unfamiliar and likely unasked-for decision-making roles on families and carers may be significant, particularly if they are already wrestling with grief and guilt in response to their situation (Hennings et al., 2010; Forbes et al., 2000). These processes, unsurprisingly, can also be difficult for people with dementia who often have a sustained wish to be more involved in the decision-making processes (Hamann et al., 2011; Tyrrell et al., 2006). The extent of this interest can also be a surprise to family and carers who know them best, as demonstrated in a study where 92% of persons with mild to moderate dementia wanted to be involved in decisions about treatment, many more than the 71% their carers anticipated would want to be involved (Hirschman et al., 2005).

Decision-making processes are complicated and don't just involve people with dementia and family members. When decisions are health-focused or the need for decision-making comes up when a person is being cared for in hospital or in an aged care facility, many types of clinicians tend to become involved in a variety of ways. A lot of the research work into this space reflects a hierarchical medically-led view of decision-making within healthcare and tends to focus on decisions in response to specific illness milestones, like decisions for specific treatments or decisions about where a person with dementia should be discharged to from hospital. As you'd expect then, doctors are the most frequently studied group within the literature on healthcare decision-making in dementia. The role of doctors has been explored in multiple types of decisions including: when to use or cease particular treatments for dementia or its symptoms such as with cholinesterase inhibitors (Franz et al., 2007); when to use or cease treatments for dementia complications or other chronic conditions happening alongside dementia, such as using antibiotics, artificial hydration or nutrition or dialysis (van der Steen & Volicer, 2011; Pasman et al., 2004; Spike, 2007); approaching or initiating end of life care in dementia (Congedo et al., 2010); initiating admission to hospital (Helton et al., 2006), or in revealing the diagnosis of dementia itself (Karnieli-Miller et al., 2007). Doctors are seen as having an important role in supporting decision-making through communicating options and information to people with dementia and their networks, while also being clinical decision-makers who make decisions about what treatments are available (Pasman et al., 2004) (Spike, 2007). Whether the role of a doctor is to support a process where a patient themselves decides or whether it is to decide on what treatments will be offered is a complicated and contentious space regardless of whether a person has dementia. However, in countries like Australia, there's general legal and ethical agreement that healthcare providers (including doctors) aren't obligated to provide a treatment that they feel is inappropriate even if they're asked to do so. So, outside of an emergency, doctors have a role in determining what treatments are appropriate for a person's situation and then in supporting a person (or the person or people who are empowered to make decisions on their behalf — see below) to make an informed decision on whether they want to proceed with whatever treatments are on offer.[11]

Doctors aren't the only healthcare providers who have a role in decision-making in dementia. Other clinicians, such as nurses, aged care workers, and allied health practitioners are also routinely involved in decision-making (Modi et al., 2007; Healy, 2000). However, it's less clear *how* they should be involved in decision-making in dementia, how comfortable they are with their involvement, and how sanctioned this contribution is as part of their role. For instance, some studies of aged care facility staff have shown that while they believe they could valuably contribute to decision-making in dementia, they also avoided involving themselves in these sorts of discussions because they felt that they lacked knowledge, authority or moral agency (Lopez et al., 2010). Clinicians' contribution to decision-making in dementia seems to vary significantly based on context including a wide variety of patient and situation specific factors (Healy, 2000). What seems like the right or best decision from clinicians' perspectives can change depending on issues like the anticipated prognosis of a person with dementia (van der Steen et al., 2009); how experienced the clinician feels in dementia care (Helton et al., 2011); the role they feel they have in decision-making (Franz et al., 2007); what sorts of decisions are being made (van der Steen et al., 2005); clinician's own history, culture and beliefs (Hinkka et al., 2002); and the rules and norms where this is all occurring (Richter et al., 2001; Helton et al., 2006). Perhaps unsurprisingly, doctors, other clinical staff, patients, and families do not always agree on what to do and an approach to manage differences in opinion can be very important (Rurup et al., 2006; Coetzee et al., 2003).

So, practically speaking, much decision-making in dementia seems to occur within some sort of process involving multiple people and requiring a consensus for a result. A shorthand for these sorts of processes in healthcare terms is shared decision-making. The idea of shared decision-making is that healthcare decisions need deciders (like patients) and people who know the options (like clinicians) to work together to explore what is available, what the implications of choosing this or that might be, and how it might fit with what's important (like a patient's values, goals and preferences) in making a decision. However, the extra level of complexity when we're talking about a person with dementia is that they may no longer be able to be fully involved in these sorts of shared decision-making processes.

Who can decide?

What should we do when a decision is required but we're not sure the person at the centre of it is able to make this decision due to their declining health? This is actually a fairly common problem. Decision-making changes in dementia for a variety of reasons. There's been a lot of work done to investigate decision-making in dementia and the perceived differences in decision-making accuracy or appropriateness relative to "normal" decision-making as measured using psychological instruments. Changes are often observable in multiple domains, including changes to memory (amnestic changes), change to risk assessment, planning, limitations to being able to perform two tasks at the same time, social cognition, and moral framing on validated test instruments (Torralva et al., 2000; Logie et al., 2004; Delazer et al., 2007; O. C. Okonkwo, Griffith, Belue, et al., 2008; O. C. Okonkwo, Griffith, Copeland, et al., 2008; Ha et al., 2012). [12]

Decision-making capacity or "capacity" is a key concept here and relates to legal and clinical frameworks used to determine a person's ability to make decisions. Capacity seems a natural extension of a rationalistic notion of autonomy in many ways. If the primary aspect of autonomy is a person's ability to make a decision that seems rational, then there needs to be some practical way of assessing this and then doing something about it if there are concerns. While determining that a person doesn't have capacity limits individual "freedom" (another important quality in rational individualist ideas of autonomy) that might be less of a problem in this situation, as the primary issue is that the person may not have autonomy (and therefore doesn't require a "normal" amount of freedom). It's also been argued that questioning capacity can, counter-intuitively, be considered as a measure of respect for its value, in that assessing capacity properly takes time and effort and so investing that time and effort indicates the value attributed to a person's autonomy (Barbas & Wilde, 2001; Darzins & Molloy, 2000). Taking the time to assess capacity properly often involves a person being tested in four cognitive domains: understanding specific situations and basic information about choices; evaluating reasonable implications or consequences of available choices; using reasoned process to weigh the risks and benefits of such choices; and communicating relatively stable and consistent choices (O'Neill & Peisah, 2011).[13] There are also multiple tools or psychometric assessments that are sometimes used to assess capacity, although considerable variation exists between the use of these tools and expert clinical assessment — and clinical assessment is usually considered the best approach in clinical (non-research) settings (Karlawish et al., 2005). People don't lack capacity just because they have dementia. However, it is true that people with dementia are more likely to lose capacity over time (Huthwaite et al., 2006; Okonkwo et al., 2007).

Despite the conceptual importance of capacity, current approaches to defining and assessing capacity may, unfortunately, harm persons with dementia. Capacity is assumed to be present unless it's assessed to be absent, so the very act of wondering about capacity (as a clinician) implies a suspicion that you won't find it. How best to use the knowledge that a person who does lack decision-making capacity is also not always clear. While decision-making capacity sounds like a general description, it's best thought of as relating to a specific decision, made by a person at one particular time. That is, a capacity assessment indicating that a person doesn't have capacity to make a real and necessary decision at a particular point (like the decision to change a will) doesn't mean that the person could never make that decision, just that they can't do so now. But in practice, reassessing capacity for different decisions at different points can seem an unattainable ideal, and so blunter and more efficient "all or nothing" approaches to decision assessment are often adopted. Capacity assessments can also, somewhat perversely, be seen as the most important thing to decide when capacity is in question when, instead, the most important decision is the decision that has led to a person's capacity *being assessed* (Bowman, 2008).

Determining that a person doesn't have capacity is only potentially helpful if that information is going to lead you to do something differently. In countries like Australia what happens next is usually the implementation of surrogate decision-making. A surrogate decision-maker can be someone who has been appointed for this role by the person prior to their losing capacity to do this (sometimes called an "enduring power of attorney") or a person appointed by a legal process when a decision is made and there isn't a decision-maker in place for a person who's lost their decision-making capacity (sometimes called a "guardian").[14] This approach of deciding that a person has lost capacity and then tapping someone else on the shoulder to make their decisions for them gets things decided, but it doesn't really achieve anything else. It doesn't, for instance, help us know how to continue to include and involve a person who may almost have capacity or has fluctuating capacity in their decisions, or how to honour their preferences if they don't align with other considerations. Persons with dementia are at particular risk of having their needs overlooked, as it's often assumed that people with dementia don't have capacity (Gallagher & Clark, 2002). These assumptions add to the yawning power differences between the clinician and the person with dementia. It is the clinician who determines that sufficient concerns are present for a capacity assessment to be warranted, and they also perform the assessment that may result in a restriction of rights. This can all become highly adversarial, as Bowman notes, where the legal framework requires that "someone will prevail in the quest to make decisions", thus setting the scene for conflict in situations where there are significant differences in views among people with dementia, potential surrogate decision-makers and clinicians regarding the need for assessment or the decisions themselves (Bowman, 2008). Legal revision and increasing oversight by empowered legal bodies (such as the Mental Health Tribunal in Victoria, Australia) has had an impact on some of these concerns for persons with mental health diagnoses; however, the determination of "incapacity" in dementia remains comparatively under-regulated and usually occurs following assessment by a single clinician (Stewart, 2006).

But it is important to note that this isn't the only model of what could or should be done next if a person with dementia's decision-making seems to have deteriorated. There's a concept called supported decision-making which can sometimes apply. This essentially means that rather than a person with dementia (or with some other challenge that impacts their decision-making capacity) having a surrogate decision-maker take over their decision-making, a process can commence where the person receives the support they require to be able to make the necessary decisions. Using Nancy's example, perhaps if Nancy and Rosie had sat down together and talked through the issues, Rosie could have supported Nancy to have made the decision. Arguably, from Nancy's perspective, that's what happened, but legally, the decision was Rosie's to make. Supported decision-making, however, intends to keep people with impaired capacity central to their own decision-making, rather than making them more ancillary when the challenges seem to suggest that this would be best or safest. There's a lot of international ethical support for the idea of supported decision-making, but it remains a fairly new idea in dementia care and isn't always backed up by laws which make it easily usable. Currently, it's often used as a principle which informs good decision-making practice, rather than a legal requirement for how to do things.

The example of advance care directives

Regardless of whether supported decision-making is available, you'd be right in wondering where the voice and views of a person with dementia (whose capacity is questioned) feature within all of this complexity. It usually depends on a variety of legal, ethical, and political considerations all of which can differ significantly depending on where you might be standing when you're asking the question. An example which highlights these challenges is the commonly available "advance care directive" (ACD). ACDs provide an ethical and legal framework to recognise and enact — through the prior documentation of their wishes — the decision-making of a person who has been determined no longer to have decision-making capacity. While ACDs are of relatively clear potential benefit for persons whose wishes are easily understood, transmissible, and uncontested, the scenario for persons with dementia can be more complex.[15]

A key idea in understanding ACDs is the notion of "precedent autonomy", famously explored by Ronald Dworkin (an American philosopher of law). The idea here in essence is that the best way of respecting autonomy in the context of a person who no longer has autonomy is by valuing the earlier decisions of that person from the time before their decision-making was in question. Ideally, this would mean that a person could complete an ACD and be confident that their decision would be known in the future if they weren't able to express it. That all seems intuitive and fair enough. But there's an extra element to this that might not be apparent on first reading. Because we're giving decision-making prominence to the past person who completed the ACD, these past decisions seem to outvote the more current preferences of a person with dementia if they've lost capacity. Dworkin's reasoning here was that this precedent autonomy was more likely to relate to deeper (and more important) preferences than the "experiential wishes" of a person with dementia who no longer has decision-making capacity (R. Dworkin, 1993). Conflict between an ACD and the later views of a person with dementia who no longer has capacity isn't likely to be common, but it's interesting to wonder whether this might be partly because conversations exploring the views of a person with dementia may not be thought necessary if there's already an answer available in an ACD. A dramatic example of this could be when a person with dementia expresses strong current preferences which are out of step with their previously stated wishes on an important topic, such as whether to accept life-prolonging treatment. In these sorts of situations, the person with dementia struggles to be heard over their own historic self whose decisions are often easier to interpret, more legally credible and (perhaps) closer to the moral judgements that those around the person with dementia now think is the decision in their "best interests".

Ironically, privileging the views of an autonomous, precedent self of a person with dementia does not prevent this past self from also being ignored. Evidence demonstrates that even if the wishes of a person with dementia are known, documented and acknowledged to be important by all involved, family and clinician preferences are still the primary factors which influence end of life choices (de Boer et al., 2010). Some would also contend that, at the point that a person with dementia loses their decision-making capacity, an ACD is no longer an "immutable" document, but subject to interpretation based on the realities of current situations, regardless of whether these were anticipated or are apprehended by the person with dementia (Muramoto, 2011). This suggests that ACDs could be seen as a communication tool that aids the interpretation of preferences rather than as specific instructions that should be followed, an approach which perhaps could lead to the preferences of the past and present person both being taken into account as much as is possible (Moody, 1996). Furthermore, some have suggested that ACDs may need to be put aside in individual cases when a person with dementia demonstrates preferences that are out of step with their past instructions, even if they no longer have capacity (Lemmens, 2012). These opinions speak to real challenges in working with ACDs and supporting persons with dementia, but they are difficult to reconcile with the legal and ethical frameworks that support the use of ACDs. It is perhaps for this reason that ACDs are often seen by families and clinicians as more theoretically than practically useful (de Boer et al., 2010). Better and more flexible mechanisms continue to be needed to support persons with dementia to have a voice and express their preferences, as our current approaches remain problematic.

The challenge of intelligibility

One of the reasons that the decision-making of persons with dementia seems so challenging is because it can be difficult to know how to interpret what's happening. The interaction of all the neuropathological, social, and communicative changes of dementia can make persons with dementia seem impossible to understand. They can become unintelligible to others. However, it is important to remember that this remains a question of perception. It may be that if we aren't sure what a person with dementia is saying, then that's on us: in other words, "just because the listener is confused doesn't mean that the speaker is confused" (Sabat & Harré, 1992).

The concept of "advance care planning" (ACP) provides a useful way to think this through a little more. Advance care planning describes varied processes that can provide people (including those with dementia) a voice in future decision-making if they become incapable. While sometimes resulting in a legally binding ACD (as we've discussed), advance care planning also includes the reflections, conversations and writing that formulate a person's preferences about their future health concerns, not just the written statement of a choice. ACP for people with dementia would seem to require a process that creates or supports intelligibility, as ACP wouldn't really be achieving the goal that's intended if the results of the process were unclear. However, a focus on simplicity and efficiency within healthcare sadly means that these processes don't always seem to improve how well we understand or listen to people with dementia. Research into ACP for persons with dementia reveals that most of us assume that we can't understand the wishes of persons with dementia. More studies are being done but we're only coming to understand how much we have to learn about this. However, some large studies of research projects (called "systematic reviews") on aspects of decision-making for people with dementia demonstrate that even when we're trying to get to the bottom of how and why we act this way, we don't really seem to ask people with dementia their opinions. For instance, in a systematic review looking at people with dementia's choices of where they wanted to be if they were dying (which can be an element of ACP) (Badrakalimuthu & Barclay, 2014) only one of the six studies included discussion of what people with dementia's own preferences were. This study (focused on the preferences of people with dementia) noted that the limited data we have suggests that it is the preferences of people around a person with dementia (usually family members) that are listened to for these sorts of big questions, not the person with dementia. Even when we do know what people with dementia want for themselves, we sometimes struggle to know how to deal with that information, particularly if it disagrees with our sense of what's best. In one study, persons with dementia who had lower scores on a cognitive test (called the Mini Mental State Exam [MMSE]) and had been determined not to have decision-making capacity were more likely to choose aggressive medical interventions than people their own age without dementia when they were talked through a health story that portrayed life-threatening situations and were asked what should be done (Fazel et al., 2000). In this case, the authors felt that aggressive interventions were a "bad" choice (a view that would be common among many healthcare providers), but they remained uncertain whether these were made because of the dementia, the influence of an intervention-focused medical culture, or perhaps due to persons with dementia valuing each moment of their lives more than we think we would in the same situation (Fazel et al., 2000). There's a lot we don't know. It's not always clear what influences decision-making in people with dementia. In this study, it could be that people with dementia interpret and relate to health stories differently, or that they valued their experience differently than was expected, or that these people with dementia had different hopes and fears than people without dementia or some other thing, we just don't know. Dworkin might have argued here that we might not be seeing a true, relevant decision from a person with dementia, but actually just their "experiential wishes" — something more responsive to the moment than reflecting a deeper sense of who they are. Maybe that's true, but how confident about that are we? Should there be an imaginary line (say the results of an assessment) where we stop asking and listening to people? I think a better take away message is that (whether a person has dementia or not) we don't know what is important to people unless we genuinely try to find out.

It's fair to ask, then, how we might find consensus on these big questions in dementia. Furthermore, how do we know if a person with dementia has views that are reasonable if there's disagreement? It's perhaps worth reminding ourselves here that our communities aren't often in agreement about what's reasonable. We tolerate and perhaps even encourage differences of opinion in many areas and among many populations. Should we feel differently when we're thinking about dementia? These are complicated questions that we'll come back to throughout this book. It is worth noting at this point that we tend to be more accepting that a person with dementia has made a valid decision (whatever it may be) if it aligns with how they used to feel about a topic. This is clearly the case when we're talking about ACD (as we discussed earlier), where there is documentation of a past preference of a person with dementia, thereby making the current preference of the person with dementia (if it is in agreement) at least feel clear and understandable (Feinberg & Whitlatch, 2001; Karel et al., 2007).

It may also be that our cultural view of dementia has an impact on what we see as reasonable decisions. Studies of clinicians suggests that they feel that an individual contribution to decision-making is less relevant in dementia in comparison to other diagnoses with some similar needs (such as strokes), so we need to be conscious that those determining the reasonableness of a decision may not feel that a person with dementia needs to be that involved (Healy, 2000). While experiences clearly change over time for people with dementia and those who care for them, it's an important counterbalance to our assumptions to note that dementia can and does include positive experiences and good stories. We assume a lot of negative parts to dementia stories. However, people with dementia often rate their experiences and their quality of life as having more value than those around them tend to (Burks et al., 2021). Studies of the reported experiences of people with dementia and their carers also demonstrate that good stories are common (Steeman et al., 2007) — not easy stories, but stories of positivity arising from working to find a balance and value within a time of difficult changes and discovering that achieving this was possible. Our often very negative assumptions about what the experience of dementia is like probably influence the sorts of decisions that we feel are reasonable for people with dementia.[16] Unfortunately, this seems to suggest that we are only really confident and well-prepared to understand people with dementia's decisions when their views don't change and when they seem to align with what we expect. ACD may be the best tool that we have so far, but as time goes on it may not be sufficient for ensuring that the preferences regarding decisions of persons with dementia are recognised by others. More work and better solutions may be required.

Decision-making in dementia happens all the time and is complicated. We know that there are many reasons why people with dementia aren't able to contribute to decision-making in the way that they used to. However, the current systems and approaches we have in place to make sure that people with dementia are safe don't seem to support them to be as included as they should be. That's particularly true as their condition worsens and if their views on important decisions seem to be changing. Clearly, it's difficult to balance these priorities and challenges, but perhaps there are extra reasons why we tend to struggle to get this right. The next chapter will explore the issue further by starting to look into some of the other ideas that contribute to decision-making and are involved in debates about how we understand people with dementia: namely, ideas of personhood, selfhood and identity.

6. Persons, identities and selves

Changing value – personhood in dementia

Deciding how involved a person with dementia can and should be in their own decision-making (including assessing their decision-making capacity) can have broad consequences. Dementia is a diagnosis and a label crowded with assumptions. Deciding that a person has dementia changes our behaviour toward them. It has been noted that when we give the label "dementia" to a person their wishes and preferences become areas of contest and negotiation (Chrisp et al., 2013). Once a person has dementia, we tend to assume that they now can't advocate for their own care, health and welfare needs and so these roles tend to be taken by others. Harrigan and Gillett take this a step further in suggesting that this also means people with dementia have a different status and less rights than everyone else — where "the rights the person enjoys diminish to the right to life, relief from suffering (as far as that is possible) and physical integrity", rather than all of the broader rights that we tend to think everyone should be confident about having (Harrigan & Gillett, 2009). In an often-underappreciated way dementia involves conflict around social recognition. From this perspective, the capacity assessment we discussed previously is a symbolically aggressive and violent act. In the name of protection, it revokes the social status that people have and permits "oppressive practices of care that further negate the social existence of individuals with dementia" (Smith, 2009). This is heavy language to make an important point. Capacity assessments aren't wrong or bad, and having systems in place to make sure that people with dementia are safe are important, but these systems and approaches are also problematic. How we decide who's in that box, when and why, is slippery and inconsistent, and there are many potential negative impacts from determining that a person can't make their own decisions, even if the motivation to do so is a good one.

Kitwood's influential description of the "malignant social psychology" of interactions with persons with dementia gets to the root of this point (Kitwood, 2019: 51). By this phrase, Kitwood is referring to the impact of the surrounding social environment on the individual's suffering and disability — specifically, how processes such as the infantilisation of persons with dementia actually creates disability, that is, they make dementia worse than it has to be. This is a little akin to the idea that, "if you don't use it, you lose it", except that in this case our society tends to act in ways that mean that people with dementia can't use the skills and capacities they still have, and so they don't use them and then they don't have them anymore. As we've noted, why we do this probably relates to the fear that dementia conjures within us as a cultural group. Coming back to the idea of intelligibility, a part of this fear for us is probably the fear that, in having dementia, we ourselves and our lives will no longer make sense within our society. We fear that dementia will strip us of our ability to continue to have the roles and statuses which have defined and underpinned how we see ourselves (Smith, 2009). This fear corresponds to the idea of a "social death" where the progression of dementia means that we are effectively dead for our society (holding little or no value) well prior to the physical death to which dementia also leads. Dementia seems so impossible to understand, a kind of tragic absence, that it makes it really difficult for any of us to put ourselves in the shoes of a person with dementia. Altogether, this means that, because we tend to believe that people with dementia are incapable of contributing to the direction of their lives, we (collectively) ensure that this is the case.

Considering what this might mean for someone is a real challenge for those of us who've never been in that position. As a little experiment I'm going to ask you to pause your reading after you get to the end of this sentence, close your eyes, and take a few moments to think about who you feel you are, and what you value about yourself. Go ahead, I promise I'll wait right here.

• • •

If you didn't do that and just read on without hesitating, I won't judge you, I promise, I won't even know. If you did reflect on that question, thanks for bearing with me.

I'm not going to presume that I could predict what might have come up for you but I'm guessing that some of it probably related to experiences and qualities that you feel you have and perhaps also to ways that you feel those around you see, understand and value you. In the field of philosophy these sorts of descriptions are often in terms like "selfhood", "identity" and "personhood". It may be that there's no more immediate assumption that I hold about myself than that I have experiences, that these correspond to some idea that I and others have about who I am and that all of this adds up to me being a person. Now, imagine that all of these aspects of yourself were not assumed but were in question, and that your ability to clarify your own experiences, feelings and interpretation of the world was significantly diminished. This is, of course, only part of what having dementia might be like but, hopefully, starts to give some sense of why being or being considered unintelligible is important in dementia. If we cannot understand a person or believe that understanding them is impossible, what value do we place on their experiences and their views on anything?

We'll discuss "selfhood", and "identity" a little later, but let's start with thinking through "personhood" because this idea has had a particular importance for how we think about dementia. Personhood is a term that most of us would feel we understand but it is (as are many important ideas) contested. Most simply, personhood describes a status of being a person relative to all the other things we consider as not being people. How we decide who or what counts as a person is where things get murky. Two approaches have been suggested to define what's necessary to be a person (Walters, 1997).[17] Personalism means believing that humans achieve their status and the associated right to resources through possessing capacities such as cognitive abilities and self-awareness. John Locke (a British philosopher who wrote about personhood among a great many other topics) argues that qualities of self-awareness and rationality are needed for personhood (Locke, 2015). It is important to note here that achieving personhood does not necessarily imply that we are the same person over the course of a lifetime. Locke considered identity as arising from an individual's relationship to their past, and their moral worth (Locke, 2015). This view suggests the curious possibility that an individual may continue to be considered a person while their identity might be changing, or perhaps be considered as having a continuing identity while no longer being a person. These complex and fascinating aspects of the concept of identity will be examined further on. At this point, it is sufficient to note that our identity and our status as a person might be separate things.

Another view of personhood, "physicalism", is where every human being, regardless of capacities, has the status of person and is inherently entitled to life and resources (Walters, 1997). This view of personhood relates to our initial existence as a human being and places less focus on the relevance of whether personhood persists.

Frey explores this perspective through considering the human (autonomous or otherwise) right not to be experimented upon, contrasted with the absence of this right for animals (Frey, 2005). Some animals, she notes, may have greater mental capacities than some humans, and may be considered as more autonomous. Frey suggests that human and animal lives have different value due to the common attribution of moral worth to human existence, regardless of such specific capacities. In short, humans (persons) deserve different treatment because they are a special case and are distinct from other non-human beings.

Further complicating matters, personhood is not always seen in such binary terms. Personhood, and the status of those being scrutinised, is sometimes seen as a continuum that's affected by the values we have as a society. Frey's suggestion that animals have less moral worth than humans arises from a frequent (but by no means universal) societal sense that animals' lives are of lower quality than humans'. From this perspective human lives are worth more than animals' lives as they share a "richness" of "content" despite the potential for variation among individual people (Frey, 2005). A continuum of personhood has also been described when comparing human experiences. Walters described a "proximate personhood", where personhood and worth are higher for those closest to "normal" (Walters, 1997). Walters' sense of "normal" relies on three capacities: the potential to develop capacities that represent a beneficial life; our development towards being such a person; and our social bonding with others and our society. The suggestion here that personhood can emerge over time introduces flexibility but defining the "normal-enough" capacities that are required for a status that's approaching personhood seems risky. The context for Walters' view is that he sought to define personhood and its socially sanctioned limits in order to make decisions about rights to life a little easier. Whether we as a social group should decide by majority or consensus who counts as a person and who doesn't is even more treacherous terrain (Fleischer, 1999). There have been many ideas of what attributes might be considered as counting towards personhood. Many have recommended that rational cognitive characteristics should be central to deciding who's in and who's out, which is clearly important when our main focus in this book is people with dementia. It's also worth noting that our social and cultural views on these things can change and that those at risk of being under scrutiny are clearly at risk of being found wanting by those doing the judging. Societies have decided in the fullness of time that what was previously thought of as "normal" approaches to valuing the status of people were actually deeply immoral. Our collective history of exclusion and poor treatment of those (such as the First Nations peoples in my home country) deemed to have characteristics or capacities which separated them from "normal" people highlights this point. If a person's status is something that must be earned or proven, then privileging those seen as "normal" is an expected result (Meilaender, 1995).

Being person-centred

Considering whether personhood might be present or absent for anyone including people with dementia is a high stakes game. However, it's also become clear that highlighting the challenges to the personhood of people with dementia has important ramifications for care practices. "Person-centred care" was a concept initially described as a way of conceptualising interactions within psychotherapy (Rogers, 1995). This language and its underlying ideas were championed by Tom Kitwood, an academic psychologist, and are now central to what we think is the best way to provide care for persons with dementia. Kitwood felt that our society's approach to personhood, which he argued had become excessively bound to the concepts of autonomy and rationality in the West, had a significant and detrimental impact on how people with dementia were recognised (Higgs & Gilleard, 2016; Kitwood, 2019). What was needed, from his perspective, was to recognise and renew personhood in dementia. Deeply important to Kitwood's view was the relationship he saw between how we regard people with dementia, the support we provide to them to continue their participation in society, and ultimately how significant the impact of their condition was on their lives. As we've noted, Kitwood argued that the loss of self that he considered to characterise dementia was exacerbated by the "malignant social psychology" of those around them, that is, the experience of dementia is in large part shaped by the expectations and behaviour of others (Kitwood, 1997, 2019). This means that the effects of the dementia, and the changed approach to social interaction from those around them contributes to a "dismantling" of self in the person with dementia (Morton, 2001). Kitwood argued that embracing a broader understanding of personhood (including that all humans have the same worth) would allow people with dementia to be regarded as maintaining their personhood — one that might increasingly be changed but was not lost (Edvardsson et al., 2008). Personhood, from Kitwood's perspective, is a status "bestowed" by others within the context of relationships and social presence (Kitwood, 2019: 7). Recognising that people with dementia continued to be people, therefore, not only restored an important status to them but also acted as a kind of "treatment" for dementia since it influenced both the experience and course of the condition.

As we've already discussed, personhood can have metaphysical aspects (e.g. in relation to the notions of self, identity and agency) and moral implications (e.g. the notion of the equal value of all persons) (Hennelly et al., 2021; Higgs & Gilleard, 2016). Kitwood's notion of personhood was simple in the sense that it focused primarily on the mutual recognition of the value of people, without particularly trying to figure out what was required for this to occur. However, its simplicity does not mean that it is problem free. If personhood is a "bestowed" status, as Kitwood thought, we might wonder (as many have) when that status should and should not be bestowed. Similarly, if we think personhood is a status which people with dementia all have, there seems less incentive for others around a person with dementia to support and maintain the capabilities that might help express a person's personhood. The person with dementia always has personhood and those around them determine that, so why should they go the effort of supporting a person with dementia to exercise and express their personhood? Additionally, while Kitwood clearly sees personhood as a changing and dynamic experience, he also thought that understanding people with dementia and providing the best care meant trying to know who the person was. This involved "maintaining," by holding "in place", an identity that has been damaged (Kitwood, 2019: 75). These are valuable goals but they also hold the seeds for further problems that come back to the issue of intelligibility. If we hold the past identities of a person with dementia as central (as Kitwood suggests we should) we create the potential for clinging to a static sense of who a person with dementia *was* at the expense of recognising who they have become and what they need and feel now.

Kitwood's person-centred care was part of a broader social mission such that: "(d)ementia would not turn out to be such a tragedy, and dementia care not so great a burden ... Rather, it may become an exemplary model of interpersonal life, an epitome of how to be human" (Kitwood & Bredin, 1992). Kitwood's hope (which I deeply but humbly echo) was that uncovering the humanity we share with people with dementia may be an important step for enhancing our ability to recognise our shared humanity and act more humanely more of the time.

While Kitwood's work relating to personhood has spurred new approaches to thinking about dementia, it is questionable whether these ideas alone can solve the problems to which dementia gives rise, and the fact that we're continuing to think this through more than twenty years after Kitwood's remarkable contribution to dementia care seems to suggest the same point.[18] While the person-centred approach is openly discussed and adopted, it is unclear whether it has been successful in moving from rhetoric to having a genuine impact on care (Packer, 2000). This may in part be due to the success of the "person-centred care" message — where the widespread use of its language has led to "woolly" assumptions of what the term means and a lack of coherence between the theory, the policy, and the care practices (Brooker, 2004). More fundamentally, however, it remains questionable whether the "answers" personhood and person-centred care provide sufficiently respond to the challenge of dementia, and whether we have yet learned the lessons that Kitwood suggested we need to learn.

Decisions, identity and selfhood

Decision-making, how it happens and what it means relate to more than just personhood. Understanding autonomy and its expression through decision-making requires us to think through other important (and related) concepts like "personal identity" and "selfhood". These terms are rich, contested, and (depending on the definition) can seem to overlap with what we've already said about personhood. In defining her notion of personhood, American philosopher Hilde Lindemann employs the metaphor of an actor on stage (Lindemann, 2014).[19] Personhood from this perspective is the character being played and the role recognised and engaged with by the crowd witnessing a performance. Identity emerges from this character role in the interplay between actors. The actors (all of us) "hold on" to these characters we play through our performance, adhering to a shared social script and responding to each other's cues. When an actor denies the cues of another character that identity is "let go" and left to travel without the ongoing support of the performance's shared narrative. This implies that our identities are stories that we shape along with others, stories in which we might be the "narrator and the main character, but ... not the sole author" (Zahavi, 2005: 180). The self, then, is the actor and effect of our unique bodily choices, senses and experiences shaped by the social norms, expectations and practices in which it participates and from which it can't be separated (Lindemann, 2014:16). This description highlights an important aspect of selfhood (with significant relevance for people with dementia) as self-experience. An experienced sense of "mineness" fundamental to all aspects of what I experience of my world, and uniquely tied to my body from which I invariably see and participate in my world (Fuchs, 2017). Our experience is inseparable from our foundational experience of ourselves (a "self-givenness"). This "mineness" experience is present when and before I turn my mind to what my experiences feel like and who it is that is having them (Zahavi, 2005). If we accept this account of identity, then selfhood and personhood are separate but clearly interrelated, shifting and responsive ideas and experiences which are not solely personal or social, but both.

Thinking a little more about what it means to have a "shifting" identity seems important at this point. Identity can sometimes be defined as a continuity, that it is the continuity of our physical body and/or of our psychological self, with its memories and mental qualities, that defines identity. The idea of a continuous identity seems to suggest something that is unchanging and persistent as a key aspect of this part of our selves. As we've already discussed, however, the notion of persistent physical or psychological aspects of our selves as the key to identity and the associated status of remaining "me" is problematic when considering conditions like dementia where progressive change is predictable and unavoidable.

Of relevance to exploring this problem is British philosopher Parfit's description of identity. Parfit, like others, thought that there was something about our psychological continuity that seems critical for the identities we experience (Parfit, 1984). But his take on this is interesting. He felt that, while personal identity seemed to entail a genuine equivalence (that I am the same as myself regardless of at what point or from what perspective this is being assessed), he also suggests that this psychological continuity could theoretically be true across more than one self.[20] Parfit's eventual position here is that, due to such problems, identity is not a practically relevant concept. The key relevant fact for

Parfit is that we have a persistent sense of psychological continuity, and connectedness. Maybe some of our worry about whether identity is the same or different is unnecessary or even missing something important. Philosopher Paul Ricoeur's notion of the different types of identity provides an additional useful angle here. Ricoeur felt that identity includes both a notion of something which remains the same, and a notion of something which results from our experience of ourselves and our examination of ourselves (Ricoeur, 1995): I am the same person at different points not because I am completely unchanged, but because on reflection and experience I have the same self-understanding, I feel that I remain the same identity, the same me. This corresponds well with Lindemann's analogy of the actors, where the actor who feels they continue to be connected to the role they are playing (and, from her more socially focused view, continues to be "held" by the others around them) continues to play the same coherent part as a persistent but changeable identity.

Bringing these ideas back to people who are involved in decision-making in dementia, it's notable that some have argued that dementia's impact on psychological states means that a deep connection between a past and future self is uncertain (Shoemaker, 2015). As we've noted, if that's true, then perhaps we should reconsider how we've used ACP and ACDs to strike a decision-making balance in dementia — as, without continuity over a lifetime, past choices may not indicate future preferences. If we go a step further and believe that a person with dementia isn't the same person they used to be, why should that past person be able to speak for this current one? Even without answering that question, believing that the past preferences of a person with dementia should outweigh their more current ones highlights what we tend to value in people (Dworkin, 1993). What we seem to do, in essence, is decide that because a person with dementia shares the same physical identity with the (autonomous/historical) former self of their past, it is that past self that is real and should be listened to rather than who they are and how they might feel *now*. Identity — autonomy — is preserved and respected through potentially devaluing or ignoring the current preferences and experiences of the person with dementia, the one most affected by the results of any decision.

An element still missing in all of this complexity derives from our having been talking about *big* decisions in our discussion up until now. Most discussion of decision-making in dementia is focused on decisions which I call milestone decisions, ones which have a large flow-on impact on what's done next. These include things like deciding whether to move to an aged care facility for instance. Most decisions aren't like that. I decide things all the time, like having a second cup of tea in the morning, and it's accurate to say that this decision is unlikely to have a lot of flow-on implications for anyone. Decision-making includes all sorts of things, and our decisions (even the very small ones) are a key aspect of the architecture of our lives, influencing what and how we experience personally and how we are experienced socially. It's also been suggested that changing life experiences for persons with dementia means that these small ("experiential") decisions are even more important expressions of self than for other people (Dresser, 1995). This phenomenon invites us to wonder how practically relevant "critical interests" are for the decisions of people with dementia. Their decision-making doesn't usually revolve around "life-changing, one-off events requiring a definitive decision, but with the daily demands of preserving dignity, maximising independence and adjusting to change" (Bowman, 2008). Even if we struggle with how involved people with dementia should be in decision-making, we shouldn't fool ourselves into thinking they don't participate in it. Decision-making continues to happen and continues to feel very important for exploring and declaring who people with dementia see themselves to be. In the words of one person with dementia, continuing to be involved in decision-making was akin to standing up and declaring, "I am still here". Their involvement in decisions supports persons with dementia to be present and to be regarded as relevant: they are both selves and persons (Fetherstonhaugh et al., 2013). In dementia, decision-making expresses to others how a person with dementia perceives themselves. These "others" around a person with dementia are important as they're often needed for decision-making to be set in motion and for decisions to be recognised. But interestingly, decision-making may also act as a process of testing the personal validity of that identity, of assessing whether, through the act of expression, the identity still fits the person with dementia. Seen in this light, people with dementia are engaged in an ongoing process of self-discovery when they're involved in decision-making, an act that includes and requires those around them. Decision-making in dementia (as it is for everyone) can't be separated from the "self", as decisions are a key part of how our selves are negotiated within the messy, connected world we live in and experience.

A new page in a story

When an actor is on stage, they are playing a part which the audience participates in believing, accepting and supporting. But the actor and the character are also different participants in the story that is being told and experienced. Stories (say of an experience of having dementia) are told and understood within societies that have their own ways of making sense of what's being shared. Our lives can be viewed as happening within moral frameworks which are socially determined and include ideas about what it is to be a person and by what mechanisms we judge success (Taylor, 1989).[21]

Stories aren't the work of individuals, they are owned and shared by communities. Additionally, the intelligibility of a person's actions within society is only determinable through understanding the broad context of their lives (MacIntyre, 1981).[22] Our stories involve decisions and events, and it is difficult to make sense of these mid-way through. Stories make best sense if we hear as much of them as is available, and the person who arguably knows the biggest part of my story is me.

Using the language of "stories" might be a little different to the language of identity or selfhood, but there are useful relationships. Studies have helpfully explored how dementia affects stories and whether people with dementia feel a sense of "narrative unity" with their own experience over time. People with dementia's responses to change and the need for decisions to be made have shown that they experience a continuity of their beliefs and that their decisions make sense within the context of their lives and express their sense of ongoing core elements of self, such as deeply held values (Menne et al., 2002). Decision-making acts as a new page in the story of a person with dementia as an expression and a reaffirmation of their selfhood.

Decisions are part of the story that expresses who we are, but we're clearly not the only characters or the only ones who are sharing these stories. Stories are told and in the telling they are interpreted. Even if we consider this book so far, I've shared a number of stories and now they're yours, something that you've thought about and might share in your own way. We all contribute to how these stories are interpreted, understood and retold, we are impacted and changed by the stories we encounter. This is because the generation and sharing of our stories is powerful work. Stories represent, shape, and simultaneously result from our experience of our world: "Stories enact realities: they bring into being what was not there before" (Frank, 2010b). Stories uncover or "make narratable" elements of how we view individuals in our society (Bérubé, 1996). Bérubé notes that it is harder to tell stories about his child who was born with Down's syndrome — and realises that *not* telling these stories is akin to admitting that there is nothing noteworthy to say. Categorising people with illness through stories can injure, but silence can do just the same (Frank, 2010b). Without the story, the life itself is invisible. The importance of this for persons with dementia cannot be overstated as this "narrative voice" is "a claim for social recognition and personhood" (Burke, 2007).

The narratives of persons with dementia, the accounts of their lives, are often held by others. This exposes to what degree these stories live between people (they're inter-subjective), rather than being possessed by a single person. Dwelling on what this means in the case of dementia "raises inescapable questions about the way we conceptualise the boundaries between self and other" (Burke, 2014). Narrative is for cultural theorist Lucy Burke an exploratory inroad into these questions, just as it is a key element in defining a self for philosopher Alasdair MacIntyre. But a focus on narrative and inter-subjectivity also exposes huge questions associated with an illness like dementia. Understanding something, like a story, to be something that lives between two people seems to suggest that they're both aware of that. But what if we can't be confident of that, such as when a person has advanced dementia. What if the person with dementia can no longer contribute to our shared story of their life and their identity? Where does the story belong then, and what does it mean? Where does the self reside when individuals are no longer able to frame their identity as a question? Harking back to the consideration of precedent autonomy and ACDs, which self is still present and being listened to if the person with dementia is no longer able to recognise themselves in the decisions that they've previously made?

Deeper selves

Different modes of considering the meaning of self-experience and selfhood in dementia may give some kind of response to these big questions. There's also an extra level to explore that might help to tie some of these thoughts of identity, selfhood, personhood and narrative together. As we have briefly mentioned before, something intrinsic here could be a quality of selfhood of a persisting "mineness" of my experience in relation to the world (Summa & Fuchs, 2015).

Importantly, this doesn't require a language or a story, it's a self-feeling of being in my experience, being in my body at this particular moment. This relates to a "body memory", a knowing how I move and do things that are meaningful and important to me, a bodily knowing of my environment and of knowing and experiencing that my body is among other bodies. None of this requires reflection or language, it's simply a knowing, we just know how it all feels because we know our bodies and our experiences (Fuchs, 2012). Fuchs has suggested that these aspects of body memory are fundamental to all of our experiences of ourselves in our world and are also preserved despite the advance of dementia (Fuchs, 2020). Despite the presence of dementia, we continue to have these experiences of bodily memory, and these are key to our experience of our selves and what we might be trying to express. This relates to Kontos's idea of "embodied selfhood". Embodied selfhood is an important aspect of the self that is maintained in someone with dementia. It isn't associated with speaking or thinking but is about how a person with dementia simply *is* in the world that they experience, and (if we're really paying attention) that we can tune into and detect this continuous and constantly expressed experience of being-in-the-world of people with dementia (Kontos, 2006).

This deepest part of selfhood does not rely on those around the person with dementia, nor on the continuation of language and the participation in narrative. It offers a tantalising sense of what we can say *stays* in dementia and why that's important. What these ideas don't do is help us much with the question of "intelligibility", although they do perhaps hint that perhaps we're not asking the right questions. If the persistent aspects of people with dementia are these deep and fundamental parts that don't need language, and it's from these parts that the fragile, changing and developing identity and selfhood which involve language and story shared among people emerge, then the worry we expend on intelligibility that works solely through our usual processes of language seems a little beside the point. I'm reminded of an experience I had the other day when I thoughtlessly asked a little electronic device to tell me about the weather outside, weather that I could see outside my window. The device hadn't updated and gave an outdated answer, and it was only when I noticed that I couldn't understand what it was trying to tell me that I realised what a weird way that was to try and find out about the weather. It was an odd way to get at what I wanted to know but, also, my inability to understand what was being communicated helped me remember there were alternatives. While we often focus on questions of understanding, identity, and personhood, what we probably really want to know from people with dementia is, "Are you still there?" All that we've discussed here seems to indicate that the person *is* still there. On these deep and important levels, the person with dementia is still there but they are different and harder to access and interpret. Focusing on these ideas of identity, selfhood and personhood in trying to convince ourselves that dementia hasn't erased that person leaves us in a difficult spot as there's so much about these ideas that changes in dementia, and we rely so much on language to reassure us that we understand what's being communicated. Even if we accept, however, that preoccupying ourselves with intelligibility may not be entirely necessary, and even if we feel reassured that people with dementia continue to have their own solid levels of meaningful experience (even if it is not available to *us*), a lot of questions remain open. What should we know and do to support and create social identities in dementia? How do we remain connected to people when dementia occurs and what does that connection mean? How should we think about decision-making; and what does caregiving mean in this context?

Dementia, it seems, challenges us on the most fundamental level because we don't know what (if anything) dementia will leave of us, and whether whatever's left will be valued and understood. In this chapter, we've explored the deepest core aspects of ourselves in terms of ideas of selfhood, personhood and identity and we've seen that dementia seems to have a deep impact on all of them. But it doesn't erase them. And this is perhaps the most important point: a person with dementia is a person and they have an identity and an experience of selfhood. Changes are likely to have occurred in these core aspects, but that doesn't mean that there's nothing there. There is, rather, an opportunity for us all to rethink how we understand dementia, and what we all contribute to it. There may be further cause for hope within the distress and tragedy of dementia.

7. Conclusions and challenges

As a common and progressive illness with limited effective treatments and huge implications for individuals and societies, dementia raises profound challenges. But the nature of dementia and its perceived impact on core valued aspects of ourselves heightens its impact and the sense of threat that it poses. In this first section, we have discussed several contemporary ways of examining dementia. We have explored where the term arose and the emergence of Alzheimer's disease as a primary community fear due, at least in part, to the language and ideas used to define and respond to it. We noted that our societies' sensitivity to the challenge of dementia seems likely to correspond to the way it seems to threaten key elements of how we understand and value our lives, particularly the importance we may place on individualistic autonomy. While other ways of thinking about ourselves, our freedom and our values are available to us, none have had the impact that individualistic autonomy has had to date, an impact which has flowed on to principlist bioethics, legal structures and other ways which we, as a community, determine the "right" way of responding to the challenges that dementia poses. This is particularly apparent when we think about decision-making in dementia, what it means, how we can support it and who should be involved in it, and how this notion helps us perceive the problems that result when we consider some people "normal" and "intelligible" and others not. A variety of different responses to these problems were also laid out including work on what values, such as personhood and experiences such as identity and selfhood, could and should mean in dementia. Ultimately, these ideas remain contested and even when persuasive, useful and influential (such as in the case of Kitwood's notion of personhood) they still remain problematic. However, as I've argued, the common understanding of dementia as a problem of individuals that's associated with an endless series of devastating losses isn't true. Dementia is more complex and wide-ranging than that. But our approach to thinking about it and working with it as a story of loss and deprivation have arguably made aspects of dementia much worse than they have to be.

An alternative way of understanding dementia seems to be required. This approach needs to be able to embrace the usual interdependence and complexity of our human experiences. It needs to encompass the nuance of the shared and personal spaces that underpin ideas and experiences, such as identity, selfhood and personhood; the ways that these latter are affected by progressive and dynamic changes like dementia; and the broader impact that this has on our understanding of ourselves and others. In the following chapters, I will try to outline where we should start with this new understanding of dementia in order to learn more about what dementia is and what it means, and crucially, what we can all do to help.

Research with people with dementia

In this book, we're proposing a new approach to thinking about dementia. To even consider such an idea we need to start with talking to the people who know dementia best. That is, people with dementia and those closest to them. As I mentioned in the Introduction, this book is based on research — some of it undertaken through studying what others have learned about dementia, and most of it through working with people who've experienced dementia in different ways. Good research takes thought and planning. In the interests of time, I'm not going to try and walk you through all the planning that was done for this research. But there may be some readers who might be interested in knowing a bit more about those sorts of "how" questions.

So, if you're of a mind to know more about how to approach research with people with dementia, you are very much encouraged to read on. If you'd rather skip ahead to "the answers" that I came to after doing this research through talking to people with dementia, they start in Part Two.

Part of the work and planning for research with people (particularly those who are at risk of being more than normally "vulnerable" — like people with dementia) also involves getting permission to conduct research through entities called Human Research Ethics Committees (or HRECs). My research discussed in this book was conducted as a formal research project with oversight of multiple HRECs. In considering how best to engage and involve people with dementia we were conscious that there is a variety of groups of people, such as people with dementia, who are often considered more "vulnerable" to risk and disadvantage in research. Our shared history of mistreating, coercing, and not informing people in the name of research has culminated in multiple different guidelines, reports and procedures to try to ensure that research is as safe as possible for all people.[23] However, it is also true that the challenges of getting this sort of research right means that research for people with dementia is less common than research for many other groups of people. This is a major problem, as we will never be able to understand complex conditions like dementia without good research, and we will never be able to have good research if we avoid including people with dementia because of the challenges of conducting this kind of research well.

I'm using "research" here as a broad term which includes a wide range of types of projects with different risks and benefits. To unpack the broad term, research, a little further it might be useful to introduce a few extra ideas about how we can understand research work. The most visible type of dementia research is likely to be those sorts of projects which focus on diagnosing or treating dementia in novel ways, such as the example of the drug aducanumab discussed earlier. All research is based on different assumptions about how the world works. These assumptions include ideas about how we view our reality (ontology), how we understand knowledge (epistemology), and how we use these ideas to justify particular approaches to research (methodology).[24] These assumptions should all link up or stack on top of each other in a way which means that the research methods employed (meaning what's actually done within the research itself) make sense relative to these assumptions. These assumptions also represent researchers' and our communities' values (that is, they are "axiological"). They influence what research is done, and how and what's considered "good research". For instance, if we can see that a study questioning whether aducanumab or an alternative treatment improves outcomes for people with dementia has many assumptions built into it. This kind of study assumes that if the researchers determine a hypothesis (aducanumab helps in dementia), design an experiment to test this, and then perform that experiment, then the results of this experiment can answer the question and improve our understanding of the problem (this can be referred to as a positivist framework). This sort of project fundamentally assumes that illness experiences are caused by specific things that can be fixed (like curing dementia by removing pathological tau and amyloid from people's brains). It also assumes that research and science are objective processes where accuracy and research rigour mean that you can be confident your results are "real" and able to be separated from human interpretation and values (Soo Parl et al., 2020). These sorts of questions often rely on tools to describe outcomes in simple numerical terms and use mathematics and statistics to come up with a "yes" or "no" answer to questions.

This kind of research is critically important and continues to be central to our ability to improve all sorts of things, healthcare included. However, and considering what we have said about dementia already in this book, we can easily see that this approach won't work for every situation or every type of question. For instance, it became quickly apparent in my research that there was a significant impact of values, culture and beliefs on what dementia means, and how we approach it. Also, the language we use to describe dementia influences our understanding of what it is. This makes it difficult to empirically measure and confidently assess the experience of dementia using the positivist framework outlined above. It seemed clear that there wasn't one type of knowledge that can be applied to dementia. This is consistent with a post-modern view of knowledge (epistemology) as a dynamic process that does not have a fixed "truth".[25]

Engaging with this fluid world of knowledge from a research perspective has all sorts of challenges, and many different approaches have been suggested. One, with the somewhat daunting name of 'hermeneutic phenomenology', suggests some key ideas which were important to this research. It suggests that we should recognise that our understanding arises from the interpretation we have of a particular moment in our world that is influenced by a variety of things such as our relationships with others. This is helpful for the kind of research discussed in this book because it allows us to stop trying to nail truth down to be a single, static thing that's able to be separated from people, because in trying to do that it seems we're missing the point. It also suggests that our experience of being and our interpretation of our world (or of our research) are interrelated and inseparable. This is a fancy way of saying that I am always a researcher and a person at the same time and I'm always assessing things with both hats on. This approach also tells us that interpretation and "being" are iterative experiences – repeated over and over — leading to a "horizon" of understanding, the extent of our understanding which changes as we do (Gadamer et al., 1975). It also means that we can never know everything. Our knowledge changes and so do we, so we're always seeking to know as much as we can. Working within this kind of framework does not entail a single specific method but needs a particular approach or mindset. It needs a researcher to be conscious that research is a situated act of interpretation, that it comes from "somewhere" rather than being something that is abstracted and objective and where the researcher (interpreter) and their interpretation is changed as a result of being involved in the research in the first place. This might sound complicated (and it can be) but the central idea here is that a researcher or research isn't a separate, clear thing that provides "truth". Rather, it's mixed up with and affected by what's being looked into. As a researcher, I think that being aware of this is a good thing because it means we can be honest and clear about what research means and what we're finding, rather than feel unduly confident about having simple answers to complicated problems.

As we discussed above, good research needs to have some coherence between its fundamental assumptions, how it justifies its approach and what it actually does: like a stack of plates, everything will balance best if it all lines up. This hermeneutic phenomenology way of understanding knowledge lends itself to research work that focuses on communication through language. This means that communication (usually, but not always through words) is the primary data source (what the researcher studies — often interviews with people) and as the means to make sense of data and describe the results of this process (what the researcher produces by doing the research). This type of research is often described as "qualitative research" as distinct from "quantitative" (numbers focused) research. Within this kind of framework, the researcher is not an expert determining an answer, but works with others and the data in a dialogue to determine the best interpretation available at the time. The results of all this will be valid but will also be an incomplete or partial answer rather than a complete solution. For this reason, it's been recommended that researchers using this approach should be comfortable with ambiguity as it is a common feature of this kind of work (Kinsella, 2006). This lens also helps us see the "subjects" of research (in this case people with dementia) as key contributors to this dialogue who need to be acknowledged through the respect and flexibility we show when developing our ideas and working with them. Ideally, this means that people with an experience of what's being examined should be involved as much and as early as possible when the project is being formulated and throughout the process thereafter.[26]

In translating these ideas to the research methods used for this project, some key points are worth drawing attention to. First, due to the problematic binaries associated with decision-making capacity, and the exclusionary results of this for research work (where people who are deemed to not have decision-making capacity are excluded from research participation), capacity assessments were not utilised when recruiting people with dementia to this project. This was possible as my study included people with dementia and their primary carers (usually children or spouses) who were usually either a legally appointed surrogate decision-maker (such as, in Australia, an enduring power of attorney) or the most appropriate person to provide an opinion on involvement in research for that person, despite not being a legal surrogate. Thus, in this project a "supported consent" process was allowed where people with dementia and the person who would be the most appropriate decision-making surrogate for them both learned about and consented to the project for themselves and each other at the same time. This effectively meant that determining capacity for consent was unnecessary for this project. Regulation around this point is complex and, despite Australia having a national ethical framework to support this kind of research, its jurisdictional interpretation is often prey to opaque legislation which may or may not address issues to do with research for people without decision-making capacity, making the jobs of the committees tasked with determining whether research can be conducted that much more difficult (Ries et al., 2017).

Another feature of the methods of this project was the use of an ongoing or process consent model. One view of research consent sees this primarily as an informed decision at a moment in time at which the person agrees to their participation. This has challenges for people with dementia whose memory of events may be variable and who may not be able to provide "informed consent" because of their changing cognition. A different way of conceptualising this challenge has become more common in dementia research and was utilised in this study. Here, researchers actively considered and checked whether participants with dementia were still happy to be involved in this work throughout the process (Dewing, 2008b). Not only that — and particularly for people with more advanced dementia — their assent or dissent to continue was also assessed. Assent (as compared with consent) has been defined in a variety of ways, but essentially describes the momentary agreement of the person to be involved in an undertaking regardless of whether they fully understand it. This idea has been increasingly recognised as critically important in dementia research (Slaughter et al., 2007).

Another important theme in determining the ethics of research is consideration of its risks and benefits. A stubbornly prevalent idea is that the risks of involving people with dementia in research are unacceptably high and the benefits low. This statement clearly covers a lot of territory, and the risks of an experimental drug trial are very different from the risks of a ten-minute conversation with a researcher in your own home. However, it's sufficient to say here that for most research with good, ethical research practices, the particular risks of research for people with dementia can be appropriately mitigated. It is also worth noting that there can be multiple and sometimes surprising benefits from research participation for vulnerable populations like those with dementia. While the potential direct benefits of research can be obvious — for instance receiving benefit from a new treatment or support — indirect or unexpected benefits from research are also important and may be more so for under-represented populations like people with dementia. For instance, work with other vulnerable populations has shown that being invited into research and having the opportunity to talk and reflect on your experiences can be beneficial and even therapeutic for research participants (Germain et al., 2016). The inclusionary act of supporting people with dementia to be involved in research can also support moral worth and social standing, as citizens and persons (Bartlett et al., 2018; Bartlett & O'Connor, 2007). This project was informed by these considerations and intended to value persons with dementia for themselves, through their contribution to this work and more broadly.

• • •

With this thinking and planning on board I set out to understand more about the experience of dementia by spending time with people with the diagnosis. For most participants, this was through interviews either alone with the person with dementia or with a support person. Interviews were usually conducted in the participant's own residence. For others with more advanced dementia and diminished verbal communication, this was through a combination of interviews and other methods included within a type of research called ethnography.[27] For each person with dementia, I also interviewed the people who are closest to them and who provide care for them at home, as well as the clinicians or paid carers who were closest to them. All of the verbal and written data from these interviews were analysed and interpreted. The key ideas which resulted from all of this are described in Part Two.

PART TWO

Dementia's impact and ripples

1. Ripples outward — hearing from those we need to learn from

Now that we've spent some time highlighting how complicated and contested the notion of dementia is, and how much our understanding of it is influenced by our cultures and our personal values, it's time for us to set these points aside somewhat. In arguing that dementia is complicated, and perhaps not exactly what we might think, I may risk being misunderstood. So, to clarify, I'm not saying dementia doesn't really exist, that it's not a diagnosis, not a problem, or not serious. Dementia is a real problem and has deep and lasting impacts on people. For most people who get dementia or who care for someone close to them who has received that diagnosis, dementia is a tragedy. But perhaps, like most tragedies, it has its lighter and darker moments. Maybe relegating dementia to being "just" a tragedy is a simplification.

I know quite a lot about dementia, but I wouldn't say that I understand the experience in the way that people who have lived it do. You might feel a little similar about your experience. As we explored in the first part of this book, the impact of dementia ripples outwards like a stone dropped into a still pond. Many people are very conscious of the existence of dementia and know things about it. Most of us have heard of dementia and seen it portrayed in social media or in a movie or a book, or have seen people with dementia, or know someone who is a carer. An increasing number of us will know a person with dementia, but many won't have been very involved with them. So, if someone asked all of us if we knew anything about dementia most of us would validly answer, "yes". We might have a community or social understanding of what dementia means. But in saying that, we might also be aware that we don't really know much about what it is to have dementia or to care for someone with dementia. Returning to the analogy of the stone falling into the pond, we have felt some of the ripples but we were too far away to experience the splash. Whom dementia affects most closely and what that means to them remains a bit out of our reach, unseen and unheard.

If that's true of you, don't feel judged. Many feel the same way. As we discussed, dementia has become a very worrying problem for our communities. It's possible that you've picked up this book because you're a bit interested, but also mostly worried about dementia. Again, that's okay. Many of us are balancing that same sense of being a bit interested but mostly worried about dementia — and most of what we hear about dementia *is* really worrying. What we hear is about descent into unintelligibility and disintegration and we're usually hearing from people who don't have dementia and whose thoughts are fuelled by their fears of what it would be like. People with an experience of dementia are also often silenced by what's occurring to them. Communication from people with dementia can seem unintelligible or absent, and carers may not have the time and energy to share much about their experience, even when they're given the opportunity to do so. To better understand dementia, we all need to try and get closer to it and to hear from the people who have really lived with and beside it. As individuals, taking that step closer will hopefully make us understand it a little better. But, collectively, each step toward understanding all the ripples that make up our experience of dementia may also help us know how to respond to it.

With those ideas in mind, let me tell you a little about the following chapters in this part of the book. They explore key ideas and experiences that came from talking to people with dementia, their carers (often family members who are children or spouses) and the clinicians or care workers who are most involved in their care. These conversations were mostly interviews with people with dementia and their close communities, singly and together, in different settings and contexts (such as homes, hospitals and aged care facilities), and they involved people with dementia of different stages and severity. In this chapter and those after, we're going to refer to these small communities that develop and are built up around a person with dementia and that change in response to their needs as "dementia networks". The chapters that follow don't attempt to capture everything that these groups of people talked about. At best, they're an attempt to work through some key ideas that the networks raised and to explore some implications that seem to come from those ideas. In some sections there may not be the detail that you're expecting. For instance, I could have spent a lot of time discussing the symptoms of dementia and the practical requirements of providing care. The people that I talked to did talk about these things, but in analysing what they've said and trying to figure out what seemed the most important things to understand, I've focused on other things. When I talked to people in these dementia networks, three central ideas seemed to be the most important — and the following chapters are going to explore these ideas and some of what people within dementia networks said about them. These ideas were that: there's not one single experience of dementia, but lots of things happening simultaneously (the dementia manifold); that decision-making is central in dementia (like stepping stones in the river); and that dementia affects and is affected by relationships (it is "our, not your, dementia").

These ideas are not an exhaustive or universal recording of what's important to people affected by dementia, but rather a careful and rigorous attempt to really understand what was important to the people I had the benefit of interviewing and with whom I had the great privilege of getting to spend time. These stories are not the answer to all our questions but might help us understand more about what our questions should be and why we are asking them.

2. The dementia manifold

Dementia means a lot of things and develops into a lot of things. From the perspective of people with dementia and their networks, it is not just something that happens to you. It is something that becomes and invests lives. It involves itself in every aspect of what and who you are. It's also not a single thing that happens in one way to a single person, but a constellation of changes that have an impact on many people.

Dementia also doesn't happen in one time. It's not like the flipping of a switch, where suddenly everything is dementia. It is a process that moves forward, affecting different people in different ways at their own pace. Dementia, oddly, also affects the future and the past. It has an impact on what past things mean now, and it shifts and distorts what futures could have seemed possible into new and worrying forms.

These might be the reasons why there seems to be so much ambiguous interpreting that goes on in dementia. Network members often expressed doubts or uncertainties about a whole host of things related to dementia, including some fundamental questions like, whether a person was "still there" and was communication possible when the dementia had advanced. What wasn't in question was that dementia had a deep impact on the people within dementia networks, and they felt changed because of it.

An assumed journey

As we've discussed, everyone knows about dementia. Perhaps, then, it's not a surprise that when you talk to people with dementia and those closest to them, they often express expectations about what the dementia experience will be like. People with dementia, their family carers and the clinicians involved in their care often talked about aspects of what the future would be like very confidently. Clinicians, like nurses, general practitioners and specialist doctors such as geriatricians, often described a "usual course" of dementia, a series of events, changes and timelines, which were likely enough that they felt that the future could be anticipated and even planned for based on this map — but not all of them all of the time. A different message was also expressed by very experienced clinicians. They felt that predicting the future for a person with dementia was very difficult. Maybe some things were easier to say with confidence, for instance, that the symptoms of dementia usually get worse over time, but predicting things in detail was incredibly challenging. They'd note that unpredictable events occurred frequently in dementia, and that dementia was not a single equivalent problem. In other words, each person with dementia had their unique case and comparing them was a challenge. Kylie, a clinical nurse consultant for an aged care facility, expressed this when she commented that, "everyone has a different illness" and that the key thing was to "understand the illness in that person". This seems to imply that while experts expected certain phases within the experience of dementia, often a slowly increasing dependence and a quiet, if tragic, decline, many aspects of what dementia involves are far more nuanced and unpredictable. Truly, predicting even the most obvious future outcomes and changes for persons with dementia remains an uncertain business. Outcomes studies suggest that persons with dementia are more likely than persons with some other conditions to experience a slow physical decline, though many aspects of their prognostication remain uncertain (Gill et al., 2010; Murray et al., 2005). What is thought to be known about the journey of dementia focuses mainly on changes that seem reasonably valid to test and measure. These include how changes in cognition or communication might manifest, or how much help a person with dementia might need with physical tasks or other aspects of experience. However, there's much that we don't know about how dementia impacts people over time, including what sorts of individual and network factors might influence how and when things change for them.

Family carers of people with dementia were confident that the future would entail loss and grief, both for the person with dementia and themselves. For some, loss meant their knowledge that dying from dementia was moving ever closer. Roy (son of June who had moderate dementia) felt that this was like "a slow ingestion of cyanide", invisible but inexorable. Carers also described the future with dementia as having "no upside", as being a "terrible" experience, and leaving them living in an already grieving state. Mandy (wife of Robert with advanced dementia) felt this was a liminal state of constant grief like being "half a widow". Other losses focused on what wouldn't happen now, because of dementia. Graham, for instance, talked about the loss of a shared future that he'd hoped to have with his partner Darren. He described "realising that you will never get to that point with Darren. You won't be two old men sitting in a cafe". While the awareness of the assumed future was ever present, most carers also felt that they knew that the day to day was hard to predict and the best way of traveling was, in the words of Sarah (wife to Keith with moderate dementia), being "prepared to take the journey, (and) don't try and predict what will happen tomorrow".

Being lost

People with dementia didn't just face symptoms of dementia or losses of their future. They also faced the real risk of losing *themselves* within or due to dementia. Dementia was seen as having an erosive impact on the unique identity of the person with dementia. This was described by carers, with people with dementia now being "a shadow of their former selves", or "decaying", "crumbling", and "disappearing". Similarly, health carers felt the person with dementia was "a shell of the old person", and "not quite the same". The symptomatic cognitive and communicative changes that seemed linked to these perceptions was most commonly amnesia (memory loss), but other symptoms such as apraxia (change in motor behaviour), anorexia (change in appetite), mood changes and changes in behaviour were also noticed and felt to be deeply involved.

People with dementia experienced this as well. A central concern was how confident they could be that they still fit into their own world. This worry often related to their issues with memory. Forgetting things was deeply unsettling in itself, but it was also unpredictable and inconsistent and made the person with dementia feel more unreliable (and usually resulted in them being less relied on by others). Amnesia placed persons with dementia in the challenging position of feeling unsure of what they have remembered or will remember, and uncertain what others may feel that they have forgotten.

Ronald (an 87-year-old man with moderate dementia) expressed this as both a defence and a question in noting that he doesn't remember what he doesn't remember: "I don't remember how much my memory loss has affected my living … In what way has my memory loss affected me?"

People with dementia feel they are "losing it" (in the words of June, a 79-year-old with moderate dementia) — their memory, their stories and other parts of who they see themselves as being. "Losing it" was something that people with dementia felt, but also something that they worried about being branded with when their dementia was obvious to others and was what people were most conscious of about them. June was chilled by the idea of "losing it" but, in a worrying demonstration of the reality of that for her, also felt the story of when that had happened also slipping away from her.

> "Um, someone said to me one day, 'you are losing it'. And I don't know who that was, um … I think I was possibly trying to remember something at the time, I don't know. It just seems so far back in my memory now, and I know it isn't all that long ago, um."

Losing it could also involve losing connection to parts of themselves that used to be important elements of their identity. Changes often started subtly but they progressed. Frank (an 84-year-old man with dementia) described "living in a world of retracted things" where others no longer needed or wanted him. Frank didn't feel there was as much need to make more of an effort to try and reconnect given that the likely result was just further reminders of his own diminishment. People with dementia were also lost to others in their network. For some, this came with a recognition that maybe more of that person could have been kept. Grace (daughter of Mary, a 98-year-old woman with advanced dementia) felt regret that she (and others) hadn't made more effort to get to know her mother, "… you probably lose a lot of history by not asking … (we) probably should ask people about their life and what they do, but they get too busy, worried about their own life". Even when the person with dementia remained within their network, "losing it" meant there were mixed responses to much of what they did and said. Activities which had been seen as self-defining for the person with dementia could be seen as a pale imitation by family carers. The pointless "skimming" of much loved, often read books or the "sad" attempts at continuing to contribute to household tasks like gardening were now merely reminders of what was lost. While these sorts of activities could be considered sad by network members, they could also still feel important and meaningful to the persons with dementia themselves and they highlighted how difficult it was to reconcile and discuss the different responses to the changes that were occurring.

Unsaid and untouched — the prison of dementia

Much that felt uncertain, worrying or predetermined within the experience of dementia was left unsaid and unexplored. Dementia's impact on relationships and communication has a clear contribution to these blocks and silences.[28] Some topics were described as being too distressing, worrying or not of interest to people with dementia, and so they were never broached. It was anticipated among healthcare providers and, usually, family carers that the dementia would get more severe, the person with dementia would become more dependent and that dementia would eventually lead to their dying — but these issues were rarely if ever discussed. It was often assumed that these topics were things that a person with dementia couldn't discuss or wouldn't want to, but this was never clarified. Health-carers protected others from their uncertain predictions about future decline without checking that this protection was wanted; and family carers often didn't try to discuss their fears with others or felt unsure who they should try to talk to about these difficult topics. These assumptions and silences contributed to how disconnected network members felt from each other, and their shared but unexpressed sense of uncertainty in the face of dementia.

A person with dementia could be lost, but they were also seen as separate from dementia. The identity of the person with dementia was often seen by other network members as trapped and suppressed by dementia rather than being disintegrated by it. The movie *Being John Malkovich* shares some valid, if clearly fantastical, similarities to this idea (Jonze, 1999). In this film, Craig Schwartz discovers a secret floor in a building that allows him to inhabit and take over, to be, the identity John Malkovich while maintaining his own sense of self. We learn that when Craig takes over, John Malkovich's self is imprisoned and held powerless. Dementia was often described as an additional and unwanted entity which invaded and took over the person, trapping the self of the person living with the diagnosis, and holding them beyond reach. This dementia identity was often "blamed" when things went awry, as an awkward and unavoidable persona that had to be lived alongside rather than being an indivisible part of who the person living with dementia was. In the film, a quirk of timing ultimately leaves Craig's self forever trapped, mute and powerless within the enfolding identity of another. Mike and Joan (the children of Nellie, an 87-year-old woman with advanced dementia) conveyed a similar sentiment in describing her dementia as a prison that their mother was trapped in. They could tell when they had their mother with them and when, by contrast, the "shutters were down" and dementia had subsumed her. Some family members talked about gaps or "chinks" in the walls that would allow glimpses of the person hidden underneath. Chinks could allow the briefest contact with "extraordinary depths" of people living with dementia, their "spark" that would shine through, otherwise obscured by the solidity of dementia.

The identity of the person with dementia was, in this sense, in relationship to dementia rather than affected by it. Family carers and clinicians explored this phenomenon by having separate relationships with the person, and with the dementia. Dementia could claim and remove the person if they had "gone over that boundary" and lost connection to everything. Many people, particularly family carers, therefore acted to preserve the identity of the person, while suppressing the dementia. Family carers took on aspects of the social identity of the person with dementia, in effect seeking to preserve the person as they remembered and had understood them. In this way, family members were involved in both representing this identity of or for the person living with dementia at the same time as they were fashioning it in a way that supported their perception of the person. Against the efforts of dementia to bury the identity of the person, the network fabricated their own representation of the person. This strategy echoes descriptions elsewhere, such as Parker's detailing the constructed identity of persons with dementia as persisting due to the actions of those around them. Karner, likewise, describes a social-self that is potentiated by the efforts of family (Parker, 2011; Karner & Bobbitt-Zeher, 2005). In all these cases the identity of the person with dementia is a continual project acted on over time and contributed to by many.

A prison for whom?

The metaphor, the "prison of dementia", invites more thought about who has been imprisoned. While many participants exposed their sense that dementia had trapped a preserved person, people living with dementia did not always seem to feel the same way. They often understood their experience as a "new normal". For some people living with dementia, the diagnosis was somewhat dismissed as a convenient medical explanation (rather than a true cause) of changes which were not that significant or were better explained by the ageing process or being human. Some felt dementia was something that they'd gotten used to and adapted to and so not really a worry. Many people living with dementia seemed to experience their sense of self and identity shifting or remaining consistent in a way which wasn't threatening to them. People with dementia often explored and expressed much more optimistic senses of what was meaningful to them and how much value we should place on their current experience. People living with dementia were often clear about how important aspects of their identity, such as being "kind" or seeing their lives as a success, continued to be important to them even if much had changed. In this light, the "normal" activities of people with dementia weren't so much "sad" or pointless but active and valiant efforts, "running very hard under water" (from Jenny, wife of Ronald with moderately advanced dementia) to maintain connection and live full days. It was also noted that the quality of some experiences of people with dementia was unknowable and could have positive aspects that weren't appreciated. Mandy (wife of Robert, an 84-year-old with advanced dementia) wondered whether having advanced dementia, maybe even to the point of being completely dependent on others, might not be that bad. "We don't know do we, because we are not doing it … Maybe they are not that unhappy about that." Similarly, family carers for people with very advanced dementia often felt that how the person with dementia intuitively acted seemed to express a continuous connection with who they'd always been and what they'd enjoyed. Pat, for example, sensed that her mother April (who had advanced dementia and lived in a high-level care facility) still connected to her history and enjoyment of being a dancer and performer when she swayed to music and mouthed the words of songs that had been important to her.

While people living with the diagnosis may not have been imprisoned by dementia, dementia often imprisoned others. Those around the person with dementia were often seen as the true victims of the illness, where the person with dementia was "blissfully unaware" of the "36-hour per day" effort being maintained around them. Carers (family carers and clinicians) felt that there were clear and high expectations about what they "should" be prepared to do to maintain people with dementia. This was true for healthcare providers who often felt burdened by their caring roles, while also feeling misunderstood and criticised by others. Health carers felt they were encumbered by expectations of the "success" of what they would be able to do for people with dementia and wondered where their roles were expected to start and finish. Managing these challenges needed work and an attention to balancing their own needs with the needs of other network members. It was even more significant for family carers who were often seen as carrying the main brunt of the physical and emotional costs of dementia. Family carers wanted to help but also felt that their care roles were a necessity and an obligation — they were carers by default. Family carers felt they were expected to provide care even when that was difficult for them to do. A frequent example was their trying to reconcile being responsible for caring for a person living with dementia with whom they had a long and complicated relationship history. For some family carers dementia seemed to box them into a situation where they were now responsible for someone by whom they were challenged, with little hope of their relationship improving.

Family carers were seen as being trapped by the diagnosis, as "prisoners". They often felt robbed of family members and partners who were their companions or supports who now had dementia; their time, energy and effort due to the caring role; and their hopes and plans for a future which was under threat due to the changing reality in which they now found themselves. In this sense, family carers saw themselves and were seen by others as the true witnesses and narrators of the impact of dementia. This isn't to say that dementia doesn't have an impact on people with dementia but that carers were often seen as the best avenue for understanding the magnitude of dementia's impact. This is likely, in part, due to the communication challenges as dementia advances. When dementia progresses, it has a greater impact on the person with the illness but, correspondingly, the impact of dementia on language and communication means that their capacity to express their experience diminishes. It's probably not surprising that carers would inherit this increasing role of articulating these new and difficult-to-express experiences. Family carers weren't only articulating dementia to others, they also often felt required to articulate and maintain the person with dementia for others. A family carer wasn't just responsible increasingly for caring for the bodily health and wellbeing of themselves and the person with dementia, they also saw themselves as having a role to care for the social health of the person with dementia. This was partly through supporting the person to continue to participate and be seen to participate in the activities that were important to them, such as getting dressed up for and attending Church. This was seen as important for lots of reasons including that these sorts of social activities were part of that person's legacy (tied to the shared sense of their identity as we discussed before). Supporting the social existence of the person with dementia was a way of not letting dementia win and of maintaining the identity of the person. But knowing this meant that carers were, again, prisoners to the increasing effort and responsibility required to maintain this identity. An impossible moral bind was described by Tony (who was the GP of person with dementia, Frank) in terms where carers "don't have a life, virtually, when they try to do their best". Not doing their best or seeking to escape the confines of their situation through placing a person in care were frequently talked about as options for family carers. Even acknowledging these as permissible, or necessary, steps was hugely confronting for some carers and a source of shame and regret for others at their "failure" when they had no other options. Health carers also echoed how difficult they felt it was to succeed in balancing these responsibilities, but they also felt that the responsibility to achieve this balance belonged with the family carers. This view seemed to imply that, while trained professionals felt there were no easy answers, they were also confident that trying to find those answers wasn't their problem. This is a subtle and important point. Everyone seemed to agree that the challenges of dementia and balancing responsibilities was unavoidable for family carers, that it wasn't their fault that they occurred. But, because they were the responsible person, it was the family carer's job to manage these challenges, or said another way, it was their fault that the problems continued. Family carers were then largely left to resolve the challenges that dementia raised, or to fail to do so. In light of this issue there was an unsurprising but also seemingly short-sighted focus on the part of clinicians on caring for carers. Family carers were recognised as carrying much of the weight of dementia but the focus on caring for them as they faltered seemed to miss an opportunity for clinicians to work with and help shoulder the load earlier. Many clinicians felt that their care role was to focus on family carers (rather than the person with dementia) as dementia worsened, adding to a sense that the most important and central person in the dementia experience is the carer. Because family carers' responses to being trapped within dementia were easier to understand and appreciate, a carer was often seen as the primary person affected by dementia.

Tunnelling through

If dementia is a prison, its walls are going to have an impact on how the people on either side can see and connect with each other. As we've noted, family carers often saw themselves and were seen by others as imprisoned by dementia. But extending this metaphor, they were trapped near the periphery. More central sections with thicker walls housed the person with dementia. The depth of their imprisonment seemed, in part, to be why there was so much focus on the easier-to-see-and-access family carers. People who were really close to a person with dementia felt that these walls made appreciating and valuing them and what they were experiencing much more challenging. But the walls weren't flawless. Sometimes a "chink" in the wall allowed others to visualise links to the person with dementia. In a comment, a moment, recounting a memory, telling a joke, or doing something in a way which was so "them", a person with dementia could be glimpsed through the walls. This "tunnelling through" was fuel for recounting previous moments and stories, connecting with how this expressed something real and deep about the person with dementia. These chinks also suggested that core, valuable aspects of that person remained present even if they were not always available but out of reach on the other side of the wall. These were moments of revelation for carers, going unnoticed, perhaps, by the person with dementia but important for those around them as evidence that key parts of them were maintained. Carers expressed how these moments were important for coping. Fragile moments of connection with the person with dementia supported carers to keep going and felt like a reward for their efforts to do so. The formidable prison of dementia meant that these connections were even more precious, and they felt key to carers' ability to endure and understand their experience.

However, when the wall was up and the prison intact, it seemed less clear to many that there was any value to the experience of the person with dementia. When persons with dementia were unable to communicate how they felt about their days in a way that others were confident they understood, the value of their experience was often questioned. But as Arthur Frank reminds us, people generally still have experiences and stories to tell even if they're no longer able to share them in a way that makes easy sense to us (Frank, 1995). From my research, it is clear that dementia affects how a person with the condition experiences their world. At the same time, dementia also influences how people express what they are experiencing. These communication changes can heighten how different relationships and experiences seem within dementia, as they make it difficult to share confidently a sense of what dementia feels like to those involved, what impact it is having. But people with dementia are still feeling and experiencing. They are still writing their own story but it's just much more difficult for them to share it. People with mild or moderately advanced dementia have described their world and their experience to me as "retracted", "vulnerable", and "ethereal", all of them kinds of experiences that sound far from ideal but still definite experiences. Importantly, these are all experiences people with dementia are aware that they are having which suggests that, while the walls of dementia may make it difficult for others to see the person behind them, they may do less to impair that person perceiving themselves. People with dementia clearly demonstrated moments of reflection, exploration and self-discovery, even if these experiences were constantly at risk of being missed or disregarded. The risks of these moments being missed were high for people with advanced dementia who were often unable to express and explain their experiences with words.

Nellie (an 86-year-old woman with advanced dementia) had made her children's clothes for many years. She was talking to me about the act of making clothes for her kids, describing this skill to me, a skill I definitely don't have. She motioned with her hands as she remembered cutting and stitching fabric. As she spoke, I could see her glow with pride and enjoyment as she realised that "yes, it was true", that she could show me how to do this. She re-discovered this knowledge within herself through trying to tell me about it. She even walked me through how she would do this using an old Singer sewing machine set up as an opportunity for residents at her aged care facility to orientate themselves and reflect (Chapman et al., 2022). These moments were fragile, often needing others to be present and to engage for their significance to be recognised. Patrick (a 70-year-old man with advanced dementia) had been an amateur artist earlier in his life. When I was sitting with Patrick, he would create a tableau on the table in front of him out of objects near at hand — such as books, cutlery and pens — would regard it and then adjust it frequently, apparently according to his sense that changes were required (Chapman et al., 2019). Patrick's "art" was visible and tangible, but it could only become perceptible as expression through the acts of others. Others were needed to interpret and give voice to what Patrick was doing. Without this, Patrick's industrious creating would just be "fiddling" rather than being an important expression that hinted at the unseen parts of his continuing experience. These expressions from within dementia weren't always focused on what seemed to be happening at that moment. People with dementia often related and explored their past and their future, even if they did so in terms of not knowing how to connect to these ideas anymore. They often expressed grand hopes for themselves, particularly the hope that dementia wasn't overpowering them. This usually didn't mean that they felt or thought that they could cure their dementia or get better, but a gentler hope that they would be able to live in such a way that meant that dementia was not as much of a concern as many feared. This hope raises some important questions for me. It makes me wonder what living in this way would look like to people outside the walls of dementia. If the person imprisoned within dementia had figured out a way to live side-by-side with, not trapped by, but connected to, dementia, would we be able to see that? Would we notice? Or would our worry about what had changed and what had been lost mean that the only "chinks" that had meaning were the ones which reminded us about how things used to be?

Deciding that some moment is a chink in the wall or that tunnelling through is even possible becomes heavy with implications. When talking about these ideas with people, I have found that a common worry is, "well that's all well and good, but how do you know?" It's a good question. How do we know that connection with a person with dementia has happened or that our contact with them is meaningful? I know from the time that I've spent with people caring for people with advanced dementia that, for many, the challenge of trying to understand what a gesture, a word, an expression could mean, or even entertaining the idea that it could have hard-to-detect meanings is just too much. Carers often feel that they're already being asked to hold so much. Opening ourselves to the possibility of deeper meanings within the loss of dementia can seem an invitation for further grief, responsibility, and exhaustion. For carers and clinicians in these situations it often felt easier to assume that no extra interpretation or understanding of a person with dementia was possible, and therefore it was reasonable (or even correct) not to try to extend themselves towards impossibility. By extension, we're also not expecting anything of a person with dementia when considering them from this perspective. It is worth asking who it is that's being cared for in that situation. It almost seems that in this view of dementia we're caring *around* the person with the diagnosis, perhaps back to encompass who they used to be, because of the sense that they're not truly present to

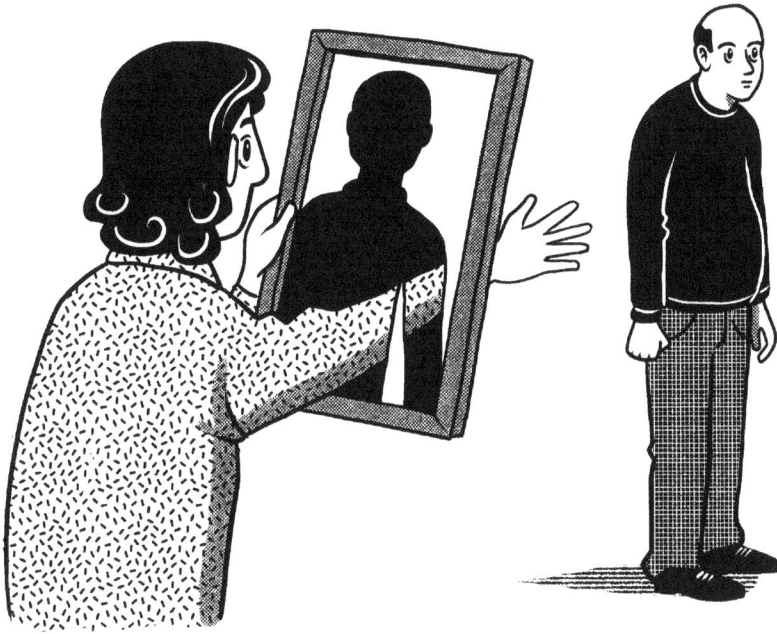

care for because we can no longer sense them. Reading one of my son's books recently introduced me to the touching work of Remy Lai. In her illustrated novel *Pie in the Sky* the family of a young boy, Jingwen, moves to Australia from Indonesia (Lai, 2019). Jingwen doesn't speak English. An Australian bus is for him a bewildering step into a Martian landscape surrounded by jabbering aliens. The aliens can't understand Jingwen and he can't understand them. The walls between them are too thick and so the people on the bus seem so unfamiliar they are no longer people. Our inability to understand attempts at interaction as communication and language is unsettling and influences how we understand those others who are jabbering at us. Ultimately, we might feel, like Jingwen did, that we have little in common with the alien beings in front of us. Overcoming the challenge of connection and communication in dementia may not be as manageable as learning a different language. But, as we've explored, chinks in the walls of dementia can be recognised in multiple, fleeting instances that do not rely on specific verbal communication, and yet can still communicate messages of the continuity of the self of the person with dementia and their connection to aspects of their identity. Maybe we don't have to try to learn a new language to connect with people with dementia in these moments. Maybe language isn't the answer.

It is important to consider what might be happening when we communicate beyond just using and interpreting verbal language. Philosopher, Immanuel Levinas thought a lot about interpersonal communication, arguing that it doesn't just happen because of what is said in language. He thought communication also occurred because of a more critical but easily missed aspect of human existence, which is that we have a very basic but powerful human connection with each other (Levinas, 1981). Levinas argued that what is "said" between people also needs the connected act of "saying" for communication to take place. This "saying" for Levinas is the connection we have with others which is fundamental to communication but occurs before and without language (it is pre-linguistic). While people create and share meanings using language, our ability to do this relies on recognising and responding to each other as fellow people without even thinking about it. Levinas felt that this responsiveness includes an intuitive sense of responsibility for other people. The qualities that are naturally part of how we engage with other people, the deep and instantaneous appreciation that we're all fundamentally alike and there for each other, opens the potential for us to speak and share (Ricoeur & Escobar, 2004). This fascinating idea seems to suggest that even if a person with dementia may no longer be able to communicate verbally in the same way, they may be able to contribute to this "saying", to participate in this mutual act of recognition and appreciation.

A man with dementia once told me that the thing that scared him most about his future was the threat of having, "no communication". Personally, I can see where he's coming from. The worry that we will no longer be understood by those whom we need to understand us is deeply disturbing. Having "no communication", however, isn't a complete understanding of the challenge when we consider this issue for people with dementia. As Levinas suggested, people with dementia and those around them may be "saying" all the time, it is just that this act isn't enough for communication to occur. We seem to be left with the *possibility* of communication and frustratingly limited tools to turn that possibility into a reality. One option is, effectively, to listen harder. From this perspective, if the possibility of communication is being limited by dementia's walls, perhaps if everyone were to focus with effort and creativity and attention the messages would get through. The common view from people around the person with dementia was that it was they who had to do most of the tunnelling. Sometimes, though, the efforts to tunnel didn't seem that well planned and could inadvertently make the distance between the two sides greater. I think a stark example of this idea is the diagnosis of Behavioural and Psychological Symptoms of Dementia (BPSD).[29] These common symptoms of advancing dementia include a range of problems from "wandering" or calling out to much more scary behaviours like violence or psychosis. These challenges were often seen by family carers and clinicians as "symptoms" and "problem behaviours". There's tremendous power in how we describe people with dementia (in itself another aspect of communication). Clinicians and carers often have the power to interpret, analyse, speak for and disregard what is said and done by people with dementia, and have a great influence on what results. Aggression and wandering could be seen by family carers and clinicians as major risks and problems needing medicines, plans and policies for safety and control. Simultaneously, some people recognised that these acts could be attempts at communication from people living with dementia who had impaired options to express themselves. Clinical nurse consultant, Kylie, noted this when she was talking about Nancy's wandering behaviours: "she was very driven, very determined to be somewhere that none of us knew where she was going. She knew and she would go there and come back". This perspective identifies this "problem behaviour" from Nancy as the expression of a preference which Nancy is not able to explain to people. Others described how some of the usual activities of aged care facilities, such as supporting showering or supporting people to be involved in events, could remind people of troubling and traumatic times earlier in their lives. Kylie said:

> "Some of the men and women have been beaten, they've been sexually assaulted, they have been raped and all sorts of things ... People who have been put in concentration camps and we put them under showers ... It does happen, they are living that. Why are we doing it to them?"

• • •

Care provided for people with dementia may inadvertently be traumatising. Inconsiderate care for people with dementia may make the problems of dementia significantly worse as broader factors than we usually appreciate contribute to what we see as problematic symptoms of dementia. Distressed and aggressive "symptoms" in response to care may be attempts at communication seeking to inform carers of the person with dementia's distress. Sometimes part of the problem with supporting communication in dementia is appreciating that people with dementia may actually be saying a lot and trying hard to be understood.

Hoping to cope

The dementia experience is difficult to cope with. People often worry about how they're going to cope, particularly in terms of worries about how hard things might be for them later on. As we've mentioned, this sort of worry is linked to an assumed future of loss and decline. A natural counter-point to our worries and fears, however, is our hopes. People with dementia, their carers and their clinicians often expressed and explored their hopes for the future, and it was these hopes that were part of how they coped with dementia's impact. The most common hopes expressed by people with dementia and carers, were unsurprisingly focused on dementia turning out to be an easier experience than had been anticipated, that the "worst" would be missed. Many people hope for unpredictable (and seemingly unlikely) events. This could include the hope that their dementia would improve or not progress, or that a treatment or research trial might become available to "beat" dementia. In these hopes, the person telling the story seemed like one of the lucky ones, a person who defied the odds. Not all stories were so upbeat, and some which expressed hope that they'd avoid the worst of dementia had a more sombre, consolatory tone. Some people with dementia to whom I spoke hoped that an early death would allow them to escape the future they foresaw. Nancy (a 91-year-old artistic and intuitive woman with moderate dementia) hoped she'd die early but also that her death would capture and express something about her life: "But I might have one final flatter, flutter before I make my exit (laughter). God knows when that will be, but I hope it won't be too long." Nancy's final flutter of artistic and empowered self-expression seemed a perfect expression of who she was and how she lived. She wanted a death on her terms.

Nancy reminds us that at least some people with dementia who hope to die feel that dying might protect something about who they are, while also allowing them to avoid becoming someone they don't want to be. Family carers reflected on dying and what dying with dementia might mean compared to other deaths that they'd experienced. Some felt that the experience of dying with dementia was particularly challenging, and would only get more so later, so it would be better for both of them for dying to happen "quicker rather than later".[30] Others felt that dementia itself may be key to a similar kind of escape. Beatrice (a 77-year-old woman with mild dementia) expressed that her dementia getting worse was a reassuring certainty: "Once it gets worse, and it will get worse, I won't know what's going on, so why should I be worried?" Some family carers similarly expressed the feeling that if people with dementia could hurry up and not know what's going on, life would be easier for everyone. Ellen (wife of Tom, a 77-year-old with mild dementia) expressed her sense that it would be "better that (they) didn't know" and explained that she found his worsening amnesia made things easier for them both. She "(gave) his clothes away sometimes without him knowing, things that he isn't going to wear" and said that "the good thing is that he doesn't remember that they are not there anymore". Tom's not remembering meant that Ellen could take charge and do what was needed, making a difficult situation slightly easier for both of them. Family carers and people with dementia had similar sorts of hopes for a range of different outcomes in which the dementia would be less of a problem. Simultaneously, though, there also seemed to be hopes for confidence and stability. Ironically enough, improving, getting worse and dying all seemed to express this same movement from one current point of difficulty, uncertainty and the expectation of change to something where the big change has already happened. It has been suggested that we can't sense and feel hope without at least some peace and stability (Zournazi & Wenders, 2013). Perhaps some of the hopes we've explored above, all of them occurring during change and upheaval can also be read as: "I hope that one day I will be in a better place where hope can be more meaningful". It seems understandable that within the chaos and change of dementia, stability, hope and peace may, for some, feel more closely associated with a more predictable and earlier decline or death than any notion of the dementia experience continuing but getting better or improving in some way. With so much change affecting so many people, perhaps the hope that things would go back to any kind of "normal" feels more fanciful than any other possibility.

Alternatively, hope may be easier to find when we feel that our worlds are predictable and stable, but sometimes uncertainty is the earliest kernel of hope. When our future seems assured and bleak it doesn't seem that unusual for uncertainty and doubt to contain a kind of hope. For some people with dementia and carers whom I've met, uncertainty was where their hope resided. Uncertainty was their antidote to an assumed future where decline, disintegration and death were the only possibilities. The hope that their experience of dementia might be different from what was expected, or that they might have been mis-diagnosed and that the term didn't even apply to them was incredibly important to some people. Uncertainty in dementia, as in all life-limiting conditions, has the potential to raise challenges and create opportunities (Kimbell et al., 2015). Feeling uncertain encompasses the need to consider that we might get worse, while also cautioning us against assuming this. In my research, people with dementia and family carers demonstrated their belief that responses to dementia were possible and, to an extent, the illness could be overcome or at least "adapted to" and coped with, with "the right kind of attitude". Despite the anticipation of "the usual journey", many perceived that their experience was not fixed and foretold, leaving room for attempts to change their experience, and for hopes for their future. Uncertainty within progressing illness suggests different kinds of hopes, for instance, the hope to live well with or despite a life-limiting illness (Kimbell et al., 2016). Hopes to live well with dementia had all sorts of meanings for people with dementia and their carers. It included growing or fostering relationships, mastering skills and crafts, reflecting on and making sense of a life well-lived, or enjoying experiences the more because of their fragility (like enjoying a good book all the more because you're not sure whether you'll be able to read it later). Some of the most important hopes to live well weren't even focused on the time that the person had left. Some people with dementia had hopes for an afterlife and a spiritual transcendence through or after their dementia. More commonly, people with dementia and family carers had more hopes for living well through more grounded legacies like passing on their life and its impact by spending time with young ones or recording stories for family or gathering to celebrate experiences together, embedding connection. For participants, uncertainty allowed the possibility of growth and change despite the assumptions that were associated with the dementia experience.

Hope or coping aren't always possible. People with dementia and those around them also expressed a sense that struggling on was sometimes all that you could aspire to. People with dementia expressed their sense of struggle with feeling burdened by changes in memory, communication, or the ability to do things that they'd previously taken for granted. They felt grief and frustration at how deep and inescapable these impacts were and how much they cost them. They often felt that they tried to do and did less as a result, living within a world of increasingly "confined spaces". Hardest for many though, wasn't the symptoms themselves but the anticipation of these problems. This could be a problem for the person's expectations of themselves. People with dementia often described the challenge of "not knowing what you've forgotten" and the difficulty of living in a perpetual state of feeling like you're not getting it. More frequent still was living with the knowledge that the expectations of others had changed in ways that you couldn't control or respond to. Ken (a highly educated man with dementia) described his feeling that what was being called his amnesia was being "entangled" with other things. He had a significant visual impairment and felt that others assumed that he had forgotten things when he actually couldn't see them. In effect, once people knew you had dementia that seemed to affect how they interpreted everything you did. June (a 79-year-old woman with mild dementia) described this as a "double whammy" in that she not only felt that she had the physical symptoms and dependence of dementia but also that she herself and others thought of her differently due to her dementia. June felt she had very little control of either of these "whammies", but just had to struggle on with them regardless. Feeling that others considered them as "odd" or treating them differently due to their diagnosis was difficult to carry and had an impact on how safe people with dementia felt outside a core circle of people who knew them with the dementia. Even in familiar circles, managing could be a struggle. Relationships were tested, seemed to involve less of the reciprocation that family carers remembered, and were now focused on an obligation to provide care. This certainly seemed true of others around those in care relationships, such as clinicians, who often expressed personal or community expectations that family carers would just do what was needed for as long as it was needed. Family carers often felt isolated with lives now subject to the changeable needs of a person they weren't sure that they knew anymore, and the judgment of community if things went wrong. Darren's and Graham's story highlighted some of these aspects.

Darren (a 64-year-old man with moderate dementia) had advancing dementia and now had quite fixated thinking and significant changes to his memory and language. Earlier in his life, though, Darren had been a senior academic and policy leader and, if anything, he seemed more connected to these roles over time. Darren spent his days writing to journals and institutions and recounting his professional achievements whenever he had a slim opportunity to do so. This was incredibly difficult for Darren's partner, Graham. Graham felt that Darren could no longer really connect with being his best friend and lover. It had slipped out of focus for him or was crowded out with bigger items on a smaller list. Too often for comfort, Graham felt that his role in their relationship was to cover for Darren's gaps in memory and his unpredictability. He spent a lot of time wondering when the world would lose patience with Darren and feeling unable to do anything to prevent it.

Carers also, therefore, experienced the double whammy of dementia's changes. Some felt that the role of caring was a process of tragic endurance. Jenny expressed this in referring to F. Scott Fitzgerald's *The Great Gatsby*:

> "Gatsby's looking across the water to where Daisy lives and he says, 'so we beat on against the current day by day' and that has come back to me now. That is how I feel."

• • •

The experience of dementia is clearly complicated, not just because it includes many aspects which vary among those affected over time, but because it is an experience that arises from many people. Dementia, in this way, isn't a diagnosis of a single person: dementia affects us, it affects people. The "prison" of dementia is both solid and ephemeral. Expectations don't always coincide with what will occur. The walls can be seen or tunnelled through, coped with, and even transcended by some. But walls they remain, and the struggle against their mute but increasing resistance or against the vast movement of the sea can be impossible. The walls of dementia's prison don't enclose the person living with dementia, as much as they connect them to those others around them, equally imprisoned within roles, challenges and uncertainties that they may feel unable to abide or withstand. Considering dementia as a neuropathological diagnosis consisting of clinical and functional changes in an individual is reductive and limiting. Dementia, as understood by those closest to it, also involves the expectation of these changes, and the responses to it. It involves the understanding of what dementia means, and how this is explored within the unfolding of daily life. This is necessarily a process that does not cease, even for people with advanced dementia, as there is always a movement towards the horizon of understanding of the dementia experience. For persons with the diagnosis, this makes them no more passengers of the condition than any other person in their network. They are the embedded nexus of this complex and changing environment.

3. Decisions in dementia
— stepping stones in the river

Decision-making is a central part of everyone's experience. From what we say and do moment to moment to decisions around major life events, much of the richness of life's content is orientated around what we decide. As we've discussed, the importance of decision-making in shaping our lives is one reason why the idea of autonomy seems so critical to many notions of a good life. From this perspective, being able to make decisions which are consistent with who we "are" expresses something fundamental about how our lives should be lived. The value that we place on decision-making also relates to why we find the notion of dementia so challenging, and what sorts of issues are identified as major challenges when a person has this diagnosis.

Decision-making is also indelibly tied up with ideas about who we are and how others see us. So much of the story of our lives is punctuated by events and moments that seem to revolve around our decisions. I decided to be a doctor, I decided to work with people with dementia, and I decided to write this book, and you decided to buy it, and then read it, is an example of a series of decisions which has led to you working through this paragraph. Many would say that these decisions express something about us, and this is where the links between decision-making and ideas like personhood, identity and selfhood start coming to the surface. There's clearly more to know and understand about you than that you are the sort of person who would buy this book but, as we discussed in the first section, the links between what we choose, what we value and how we and others see us are comprehensive. Coming back to dementia, we also noted that decision-making changes in dementia, and some people aren't able to express their wishes easily or make decisions when the condition is advanced. It's also probably true to say and is commonly argued that personhood, identity and selfhood are changed by dementia, rather than lost. However, the need for making decisions doesn't go away because of dementia and some decisions are made more complex and fraught by the challenge of how to involve the person with dementia. Meeting this challenge seems to result in a process of decision-making that occurs continuously for people with dementia and those around them. These moments and processes of decision act like a series of stepping stones that can be followed backwards and forwards across the rush of change and activity that dementia entails.

The right decision

When I talked to people with dementia and their networks it became clear that decision-making occurs frequently and is important and multi-faceted. Many decisions had the quality of milestone decisions which we discussed in Part One. These sorts of decisions were bold print, capital letter decisions where a lot was at stake, and everyone knew a decision needed to be made. As stepping stones, they rose high and were clearly visible, shifting the contour of the water's movement with their significance. Some examples included deciding to move to a new place to live due to the challenges of where they were currently living, going into hospital or appointing someone to be a surrogate decision-maker. But there were also a host of smaller decisions that people with dementia and their networks talked about, including small everyday decisions, like, for instance, deciding to go out for a walk to the shops, and their roles in making those decisions.[31] Small decisions also included really subtle things that weren't even obviously decisions at all, like the decisions people with dementia described about how they would respond to a situation, and how they weighed up and decided what was important to them now compared to before. These small decisions didn't always have a result where deciding something resulted in obvious changes (such as, for example, moving house). As stepping stones these were often obscured and hard to appreciate. But that didn't mean that they weren't important, and some people with dementia felt that some of these small and silent decisions expressed really important things about who they felt they were. While small decisions didn't always have obvious results, some decision-making processes never seemed to have a result at all. Some decision-making processes were full of questions without a result (a kind of constant deciding) or there were multiple decisions over time that led in different directions. So, there wasn't only one kind of decision that related to dementia networks; and there was much that was decided that wasn't among the milestone decisions that get the most focus in our ethical and legal deliberations. Decisions were also closely tied to the idea of self-expression for people with dementia and their networks. What was decided or how it was being decided said things about all of those involved. The person with dementia, in particular, and those in the network were very conscious that this was the case.

In talking to people with dementia and their networks there was a clear focus on the idea of "right" decisions. People with dementia and their networks perceived that there were "right" decisions that could be made and making these decisions was generally a good thing. These decisions could be "right" for lots of different reasons. A decision mght be "right" in an obvious way because everyone agreed that's what should be done. Such decisions usually aligned with everyone's preferences or values and therefore, it was just "right" to do that thing. On a more subtle level, dementia-decisions were also considered "right" if they expressed something about how the person with dementia (and others) saw themselves – expressed their identity.

Decisions in dementia were judged as good or bad according to how consistent they seemed with the roles, values, relationships or experiences of the person with dementia. A person who saw themselves as a "scientist", or a "leader", or a "mother" felt the right decisions for them related to central characteristics of their identity that they wished to express and uphold. Interestingly, the expression of identity through decision-making by people with dementia seemed sometimes to focus on partial aspects of the complex identities that a person with dementia had had throughout their life. People with dementia often seemed to feel more connected to some aspects their identities than others, and it was through these aspects that decision-making was understood. Sometimes, however, these favoured decision-making identities seemed more relevant and made more sense to the person with dementia than they did to others around them.

• • •

This leads us to the somewhat obvious acknowledgment that decisions can be "right" viewed through one lens and not through another. For instance, a decision could be "right" for one person and not another or be true to one person's view of their life and not from another's. Notably, when such disputes or differences about what was "right" occurred, a person with dementia's views generally seemed to have less status or be less effective in influencing what occurred (what was decided) and within the story of why this decision was made. This often related to changes in memory (amnesia) and communication. It was hard for persons with dementia in a practical sense to sway situations due to dementia-related changes. In addition to this, however, the views of people other than the person with dementia themselves generally seemed more powerful and important to members of the network.

"Right" decisions were often shared through stories which expressed something about the person with dementia and their relationship to their world. Decision-making stories in dementia seemed to be like a busy identity-factory, where old stories were retro-fitted and new ones created. Telling a story is purposeful, we do it for a reason and we do it because we've decided to. Decision-making stories for people with dementia therefore included a number of levels of decisions, not only what was in the story but also why was it being told, and to whom. In essence, decisions which were "right" because they expressed some key and valued aspect of the continuation of the person with dementia's identity were also more easily narratable and more readily shared. This frequently resulted in a shared process of curating the lives and stories of people with dementia to draw reference to important key elements of their identities expressed through the decisions that they'd made. These decision-making stories often expressed qualities of the person with dementia — such as their kindness, their humour, their intellect, their wisdom or their bravery. These were stories told by people with dementia and their networks to others (like me as a researcher or to other family and friends) which expressed (in the words of Frank, a 77-year-old man with moderate dementia and his family) that they had "... a life worth remembering" and that they'd been central to it. These stories expressed decisions about how to live a life, but also expressed decisions about how to share a life and an (often threatened) identity through stories. These stories had sometimes been shared many times before with a sense that others (not the person with dementia) would carry these stories and this version of the person with dementia's identity forward. These decisions involved many people and became shared acts that defined families and communities. But even narratable stories that were "right" because they reinforced key parts of an identity could be contested. For instance, Frank also told the story of a decision to go to hospital. His version of the story was that he felt going to hospital was the right thing to do and "wasn't worried about it in the slightest". This all made sense for Frank since he understood his identity and his selfhood around his faith and spiritual beliefs which he felt made him very "relaxed" and philosophical about his dementia and the challenges it created. However, his wife, Julie, then shared her recollection of that time in hospital. She remembered Frank being desperate to return home and pleading with her to effect this. Frank couldn't remember doing that and found it hard to reconcile with what he knew and valued about himself. Frank's story expressed the decisions that he remembered and that made sense to him, while Julie's story was a decision to set the record straight, even though this was distressing to Frank and undercut his view of his life. Decision-making was a powerful business of creation, perpetuation and expressing and reconciling conflicts, where what was shared about "right" decisions seemed often related to an expression of what people with dementia and their networks wanted to be understood and to continue about them.

What does a wrong decision mean?

Decision-making stories in dementia highlight what people think has stayed the same and what has changed about people with dementia, and they can also demonstrate what people want to change or stay the same. As I discussed in Part One of this book, our stories about ourselves are ours not so much because they express an unchanging person, but because they continue to feature us as the central character. However, there is a tension here. Even though I am a central and (currently) persisting character, I'm not the only narrator of my story. Similarly, the stories of people with dementia have multiple narrators. The different versions of decision-making stories in dementia shared by various narrators can strongly influence how these stories feel to us as listeners, and what they say about the characters involved. In my research, decision-making didn't always reflect an unchanged or an unchallenged story. When people with dementia's goals, preferences or decisions were at odds with what was expected by others, this often led to challenges and conflict — ultimately becoming "wrong" decisions for dementia networks. Dementia networks talked about wrong decisions quite a lot. Wrong decisions could take many forms. The following story from Nicholas and Hanna about Nicholas's driving licence was a good example.

> Nicholas was a 75-year-old ex-accountant with moderate dementia who lived at home with his wife Hanna. From his perspective, Nicholas's life had been a highly successful endeavour, largely due to his ability to rationally approach and sort out problems ("the scientific method"). However, Stewart (Nicholas's GP) had recently decided that Nicholas's progressing dementia meant that he shouldn't drive anymore, which was a hugely significant change. This unexpected milestone decision affronted Nicholas's

view of his success and independence. It didn't make sense to his view of himself. Nicholas ruminated on this point. He felt no one could explain the "logic" of it in a way that made sense to him as a "scientific thinker". The only explanation that made sense to him was that the decision to revoke his licence was wrong.

Hanna felt completely exhausted by this story and its importance to Nicholas. It was like an unwelcome guest she had lost patience with. Part of the frustration for her was over-familiarity. Nicholas's self-focus on his success and the importance of this over other considerations wasn't a new problem. Hanna felt Nicholas had been like that for years, well before the dementia. But the story of his driving licence encapsulated her weariness with his persistence and inflexibility.

Without telling him, she'd decided that the best way to make their important decisions was to leave him out of it. She'd hoped that this would mean they'd fight less but it wasn't quite clear that was the case. The slow stream of interrelated decisions that needed to be made seemed to highlight the differences between how Nicholas saw himself, as an unfairly treated "logical man", and how others now tended to see him, as an angry and tiresome, confused man who couldn't be reasoned with and wasn't safe. No one was able to support Nicholas to see the decision in a way which made sense to him, and this continued to reinforce for him his perception that the decisions being made were obviously wrong and unreasonable. No one seemed to have the tools or the energy to bridge this gap and connect what was happening to Nicholas's sense of the man he was.

Thinking through Nicholas's and Hanna's story in more detail can start to unearth how complex determining what a "wrong" decision in dementia can mean. Nicholas felt that revoking his licence was the wrong decision. He felt his opinion must be accurate because his self-description as a successful "scientific thinker" meant that his view must be logical, and that his irritation at the decisions being made around him was justified. Hanna felt that Nicholas's stubborn rebellion against the decision to remove his licence was wrong, diminishing her patience with him further. Given the relationship between decisions and identity, it's interesting that Nicholas's antagonism to the decision feels "right" in the sense that both Nicholas and Hanna feel that this is in keeping with who Nicholas is from their different perspectives. It probably doesn't matter whether we consider Nicholas's self-experience of rationality and success as a "true" expression of who he was, or something more like a manifestation of the change to his thinking and experience due to the dementia.[32] What we hear from Nicholas and Hanna suggests that an earlier version of Nicholas would probably have agreed with the spirit of Nicholas's current view of himself. It's more arguable whether he'd be keen to include the present conflict that was arising from his inflexible fixation on this self-story in his long-term plan for himself. Nevertheless, the conflict related to Nicholas's wishes and view of himself from Hanna's perspective wasn't new and didn't start with his dementia diagnosis. The decisions that were made were interpreted by Nicholas through his sense of his life and his role in it and contributed to the stories that he and his network shared about what the dementia experience meant to them.

Decisions that were felt to be "wrong" seemed more likely to be interpreted as something occurring "because of the dementia" and therefore not representing changes to a core sense of the identity of that person. On the other hand, "right" decisions were usually seen as expressing important components of a real identity despite the challenge of the dementia. In this way, the dementia was often a root cause for wrong decisions, and right decisions were considered as even more telling and important due to their occurring despite the dementia. Mandy told a story of her husband (Robert) who had dementia which highlighted several of these elements in a single decision-making process.

> Robert was a vet and was still working when he was diagnosed with dementia. He'd always been passionate about his work. He'd loved everything about being a vet and really lived through his role and profession. Over time, it was clear that his work was becoming more of a challenge for him. He also noticed that he was having difficulties doing things at work which used to be routine. Looking further into why led to his diagnosis. But Robert struggled on working, from the perspective of Mandy and his colleagues probably for longer than he should have. To Mandy's relief, Robert eventually decided that he would stop working and told everyone at work that this was his plan — which was sad but also seemed like the right next step for Robert. Robert's colleagues were happy for him and, quietly, more relieved than they let on. They organised a retirement party for him. However, soon after the party Robert

seemed to forget his decision or revised it. He wanted to continue working. This was immediately very awkward for the staff and clients who had recently wished him well at his retirement party, particularly given the collective sense that his work was no longer safe for him. A trusted friend and colleague stepped in to help Robert stay with the decision he'd already made. But Mandy felt that the confusion made a stressful and emotional time even harder for everyone, particularly for Robert.

Robert's decision to stop working was seen as an authentic "right" decision that reflected who he was, and his decision to return to being a vet was seen as arising from his dementia. However, his decision to continue to be a vet (as impossible and unsafe as this was) was equally likely an expression of his sense that he continued to identify with this personal story, not just that the dementia was eclipsing his ability to make good decisions. In these moments, decision-making often exposed the increased distances between how the person with dementia saw themselves and how their identity was understood by others. People in dementia networks usually assumed that goals and preferences should be stable, and that such stability would indicate the "real" self of the person with dementia, particularly when communication difficulties became more pronounced. When persons with dementia decided in ways that seemed to counteract the assumed wishes of their "real" historic self, the relevance of these new opinions were questioned, and decisions were often felt to be wrong. Dementia changes, particularly changes to memory and communication, undermined the possibility of a coherent single self being experienced and expressed through decision-making. These dynamics exposed tensions between beliefs about the stability of identity and participants' experiences of multiple different selves, particularly in those with dementia.

This was not solo work. Everyone around the person with dementia contributes to what results. If decisions are constantly being made and potentially filled with meaning, the potential for these to have huge implications for identities is very real. In my study, a common and important decision among family members and clinicians was what health information to share with people with dementia. Examples included whether to discuss what the future might involve (as when clinicians make choices about discussing a prognosis), the challenges caused by a person with dementia's behaviour or symptoms (often expressed by family members or carers), or particular worries or fears (like a worry that living at home won't be safe forever). These topics often involved hidden decisions within dementia networks when, for a variety of reasons, a decision had been made not to discuss something with a person with dementia and they weren't even aware this decision had taken place. Talking about these decisions usually expressed the genuine care of those involved in wanting to protect the person with dementia and protect themselves from unhelpful or burdensome pain or situations. But these choices could also feed into expectations and bolster perceptions that people with dementia were no longer able or trusted to participate in this level of understanding of their own lives.

Interpreting identity

If decisions express who we are but what seems to be the "right" decision can change in dementia, what does that mean for who we are? In other words, does dementia change our identity in some fundamental way? In thinking through this problem Ricoeur's differentiation between identity as the quality of sameness, and identity as the type of self-understanding linked to the question, "who am I?" again seems important — as answering a "who am I?" question is not a simple statement or definition but a reflection on our lives and our experiences (Ricoeur, 1995; Zahavi, 2005). So, I could be the same identity at different points not because I'm completely the same but because I feel I'm the same in some way, I feel I continue to be me.

• • •

As we discussed earlier in Part One and based on what our dementia networks have been telling us, these ideas all seem fairly important when we start thinking through dementia's impact, and they seem closely tied to decision-making. People with dementia often express how they see themselves and make claims as to how they would like to be seen and understood by others, and this tends to become clear in decision-making. Dementia clearly has an impact on this process, but it's not the only thing that impacts our access to, or our expression of, our experiences. Many of us have a fairly tenuous sense of connection to our historical selves, particularly as the years pass and as the world and our experience unavoidably changes. This shifting perspective creates a paradoxical distance between a sense of our current self and the stream of lived selves that remain isolated in our past (Bateman, 2014). For Slovenian philosopher, Slavoj Žižek, this is part of the paradox that defines the human experience, the separation of the "one from itself". [33] We are unable to see ourselves as a unity of our thought and our being, and it is this tension that contributes to the constant "becoming" of our experience (Žižek, 2006b: 7). We are, to some extent, always newly made, constantly refashioning ourselves from everything that we now have available to us. Coming back to Ricoeur's points noted above, the "sameness" element of identity from this perspective would be that we're always a work in process and always a little difficult to reconcile with how we used to be.

For people with dementia, cognitive and communicative changes make this process much harder. Changes in memory in particular make connecting to past selves, or even understanding past selves through events and choices, increasingly difficult. Dementia makes it more challenging for those with the diagnosis to weave themselves into their own story. But it's also probably fairly normal for "normal" people without dementia to struggle to connect with their past selves in a story. My brother recently recounted a story to me that I had told him a number of years ago. The story's facts checked out, and it sounded like one of my stories but, honestly, I had virtually no memory of it (other than it coming back to me after he'd conveniently told me all about it). Which self does that story belong to? Maybe you've had similar experiences? Most of us can half recall an awkward, youthful version of ourselves who made questionable choices in our past, who we probably haven't thought about for a long time and who likely doesn't easily fit into our story now. What's the unchanging part of you in your current story? We can find a more literary version of this idea in Marcel Proust's, *Remembrance of Things Past* in which a narrator shares his story as a series of interwoven, perfectly described moments (Proust, 1982). After a while, the existence of this narrator and who they are apart from the story starts to seem less and less relevant. There's just the story. Being unable to identify a single narrator doesn't stop a person's story from continuing to unfold. All of our lives are experienced as a series of pregnant moments, an array of fragile "forking paths",[34] which are ours and are inescapable (Deleuze et al., 1987). While this might all sound like I'm describing our lives as unmoored, I'm describing them more as not needing or not necessarily including some continuous or unchanged sense of who we are and where we've been in order to continue to work (Holland, 2013).

Identities just don't need to be fixed and continuous to make sense. Parfit, for example, liked the rather curious term "series-person" better than "identity" for people because he thought identity didn't really get an important point across. Being a series-person suggests I'm not the "me" I identify as myself. I am, instead, a connected chain of persons with a shared sense of continuity, experiences and responses (Parfit, 1984: 290). For Parfit, the question of whether this series-person is the same person or not is largely irrelevant. His point here is that as a series-person we remain a person and we remain connected to the other people that we have been at all of the different time-points in our life. This powerful idea raises interesting possibilities regarding the relationship between the decisions we make at any moment and what this says about who we are and how we experience ourselves. Being able to experience and express a sense of being "ourselves" at any point seems an important gesture towards maintaining our identity across the series of people that we have been. Even the simple decision to reflect on whether we remain the same or not, whether our identity has or hasn't changed over time, creates a link, a connection, with those other past people.

These ideas suggest that we may all set the bar too high when determining that dementia leads to the erosion and disruption of identity. While changes in identity clearly take place, people with dementia continue to reflect and create links with who they have been despite the progression of their condition, for example:

> Tim, a 72-year-old man with moderate dementia reflected that he continued to feel connected to a lifelong wish to be a positive person. Tim knew that he had changed and was aware of the impact of dementia on his life and the life of others. But he felt that he could still express his positivity through choosing to accept his diagnosis. Tim said, "That's probably about as good as you could expect it to be at this stage in your life. That is how I look at it … just accept that (the dementia) is there. I think the main trick is to try and live with it".

Not all people with dementia, however, feel a strong relationship between who they see themselves as now and who they feel they used to be. But, reflecting on who we used to be creates connections with who we are now, even for people who have dementia. For Tim, and other people with dementia, these moments of reflection and the choices that relate to them, can be powerful links and opportunities to develop stories and identities. Tim's decision to try and accept dementia should also remind us that these complicated links between decision-making and identity are not all about making sense of who we were. They are also central to who we are now, and who we might be later.

Making decisions is a key activity in the factory of identity generation. Before we think this through a little further, I'd like to return briefly to the concept of autonomy and present a different way of thinking about this key idea. As I've already noted, the philosopher Cornelius Castoriadis suggested that an individual (or populace) has autonomy when they engage in self-reflection (Castoriadis, 1991). He felt that autonomy is valuable not merely because it relates to how we govern ourselves but because carefully thinking through who we are is an act of self-creation. This autonomy, arising from self-reflection, is an act of questioning, of uncertainty rather than attainment. It is a perpetual process of investigation. For Castoriadis such autonomy seeks to question fundamental assumptions and acts upon this investigation, and it is through this process that our selves arise. Decisions in dementia, such as Tim's decision about who he wanted to be now, often express this relationship between how we make sense of the past, what that means for what we should do in the present, and who that means we are carrying forward from that moment. As Castoriadis suggested, this process is never finished, but neither is it unavailable to people with dementia due to the condition itself. Dementia changes how people reflect about themselves and how easy or not it is for others to appreciate that this is taking place, but it does not dismantle this reflective, autonomous self that arises when people with dementia think and wonder about themselves. It may also be true that while dementia creates the context for decision-making for those people with the diagnosis and those around them, the challenge of dementia also acts as a fuel for self-reflection, raising questions and uncertainties that need processing. It's no doubt true that these are uncomfortable and difficult uncertainties for people with dementia and those close to them to think through. As we've seen, dementia takes a huge toll on people. However, the difficult questions that dementia raises about who I am now and whether I'm the same now, as challenging as they are, could be seen as a support for expressing something important about ourselves. If we are who we are through wondering about such questions, it is in posing these questions that we start to find answers. From this perspective, dementia starts to seem like a demonstration of the dynamic, connected fluidity of our identities rather than something which fundamentally challenges or negates these core parts of our selves.

No solitary selves

A further key element of decision-making in dementia is that it occurs within and is contributed to by groups of people, that is, it occurs relationally. The simplest relational aspect of dementia is where decision-making processes involve multiple people, or where multiple people have inter-related decisions to make. However, there are subtler levels to this. In my study, whether a decision was considered a "right" decision was contingent on needs and contributions of others within the network, not just of the person with the diagnosis. When talking to people with dementia and their networks, choices were sometimes "right" because network members other than the person with dementia judged them to be the correct thing to do. In stories where network members judged what the "right" thing to do was, the decisions were often things many of us would readily agree with (such as Mandy's story about hoping Robert would retire). In other stories, a person in the dementia network's view of what was "right" was more arguable. An example was the decision made by Deborah, a carer for a person with dementia, never to ask the people she cared for about their hopes or goals for the future because she felt that, as a progressive condition, there wasn't room in dementia for hopes and goals. Because of Deborah's power in those relationships these questions were, of course, never raised. People in the dementia network had a powerful influence on what was considered the "right" decisions. Sometimes decisions were "right" within the network because they were right for network members other than the person with dementia. These sorts of decisions could still express identity and self-expression but not always in the way anticipated. The following story provides an example:

> Ken was a retired academic, a "big noise" in his time and in his field, whom I met in the home he shared with his wife Sarah. Sarah had, later in her life, re-trained as a nurse. She felt that her clinical work had been very helpful in understanding what Ken's diagnosis of dementia would mean for them and how best to support him. She was particularly aware that Ken would get worse over time, and felt they needed to embrace every opportunity to live the lives that they

enjoyed before these were taken from them by his dementia. Ken and Sarah were both charming, well-spoken people who had a sense of the finer things in life and were clearly well-liked, including for their habit of throwing lavish parties for their friends and family.

Understanding this background made Sarah's story about their last big party feel so important. It was the last time Ken had given a speech. When I'd met him, I'd been quite entranced by Ken's nimble turn of phrase. He was a great conversationalist and apparently an exceptional public speaker. He'd usually spoken at their parties in the past and over time this had become an expected part of their events. It was now a year or so after Ken's diagnosis and Sarah started to wonder about when they should tell people what was happening. As part of preparing, they decided that they should throw an anniversary party for themselves. Sarah planned the party feeling fully aware that a lot would soon change for them both. It was a wistful event they were planning that quietly honoured the lives they'd had and said goodbye to those times.

Sarah planned the party to a tee, leaving no aspect unconsidered. She asked Ken if he'd give a speech, really just to thank everyone for coming and for their friendship, and he agreed. On the night of the party Sarah felt the speech was fine. "Not his best" but Sarah felt that it wasn't likely that anyone, other than her, would have noticed that Ken seemed a little different. Afterwards, though, she realised that Ken's speech had had the biggest impact on Ken himself. Sarah had meant for his speech to act as natural expression of a key part of who Ken was for her. But Ken told her that he'd found speaking very difficult and had been really worried about exposing his dementia to others unintentionally. After the party he'd approached her, obviously worried, and asked, "Was I alright? Did I let you down?" Sarah realised at that point that, while they'd discussed and agreed together that he would give a speech, Ken had really been doing it for her and her sense of what their big party should be like. Sarah reflected that she had "taken for granted" an identity for Ken that she still wanted to keep solid but in which Ken no longer felt confident.

Ken's making a speech at the party was the right decision for Sarah because it fit her needs and reflected what the party represented for her. She only realised in retrospect the assumptions that she'd been making and that it might have been difficult for Ken to have talked to her about his own worries. "Right" decisions made by others could mould people with dementia into identities that fit what was decided. However, "right" decisions made by people with dementia could also be made with others in mind and show another type of this relational quality of decision-making and identity. The following story explores this idea:

> Julie and Frank, both with tears in their eyes, shared a touching story about the moment Frank (a husband with dementia) helped Julie think through the decision to leave their family home and move somewhere to receive more care. Frank, a house-proud man, had wanted them to live in their family home for the rest of their lives, but in talking about it with Julie in that moment he realised that he'd changed his mind. He expressed his sense that living where he wanted to had always been important, but not as important to him as taking care of Julie. He said, "Well darling, I've been very aware of the weight you've been carrying and I have so longed to be able to do something to help you, and I think this is the answer".

Here, Frank makes a decision for Julie, but it also expresses something deep about Frank's identity and their relationship. It is the connection and alignment of all of these things that make this such a right decision for Frank and Julie. The same realisation obviously helped Frank to make this decision in the first place. Decision-making in dementia helps bring to light how decisions arise relationally, how this relates to the mutual process of creation of identity, but also that these normal phenomena continue within dementia, despite all the worry about loss of identity that dementia (justifiably) entails.

Dementia affects the needs of many people, and the decisions that result from this catalyse new elements of self-reflection and expression, not just for the person with dementia but for all of those people affected by the diagnosis and the resulting changes. This sense of decision-making as enmeshed in a web of relational impacts and influences doesn't diminish the relevance of ideas like autonomy. As we've described previously, a relational sense of these values would suggest that there cannot be autonomy without some sort of influence. Important aspects of autonomous self-reflection and decision-making result from our being consciously part of and engaged with our living world and all the inherent compromises and responsibilities that go along with that and are not just limited to a personal or internal process resulting in expression of our free will (Agich, 1993b). Regardless of whether we have dementia or not, we become our most autonomous selves through our involvement in our world, through welcoming our dependence on it, rather than trying to act as though we were separate from it. Perhaps it is better to consider decision-making an expression of "selves" both in the variety of selves that a single person lives, but also the multitude of others to whom we "belong", as part of our constantly changing world (Bauman, 2004a).

Challenges of complexity

Decision-making poses real challenges for people with dementia and those who care for them. Generally, we consider the decisions that we make in life as fairly isolated and specific. By that I mean, the very word decision suggests something that is finite and concluded that we make and move on from. However, the decisions that are needed when a person has dementia are not like this. From talking to people with dementia and their networks it is clear that their decisions are not isolated or discrete but form part of a stream of choices and consequences. A "single" decision arises as a result of series of events and other decisions and leads to a variety of results, some with significant implications all of which can have an impact on what seems like the best option. Making a single decision may not be as easy as it sounds as consequences ripple outwards. People with dementia and their networks also note that this sense of the inter-connectedness of events and issues influences how decisions feel. They can also make it feel uncertain whether there are genuine choices available. Mandy's and Robert's story about deciding whether to go to hospital is an example:

> Mandy lived at home with Robert her husband of many years whose dementia was getting worse and worse. Mandy had made a decision long ago that she didn't want Robert to be given medicines to control his sometimes agitated and confused behaviour. Nevertheless, she felt like she was in a terrible bind. She wasn't sure that staying at home together was safe anymore. He really needed care all of the time. He now wandered at night and didn't always make it to the bathroom. The combination of the care load that she carried and her sleeplessness was making it very difficult for her to face each day. The only alternative seemed to be Robert's going to hospital. But Mandy felt that if he did go to hospital (and likely,

ultimately, to somewhere like an aged care facility) he almost certainly would be more agitated, and they would want to give him these medications. Mandy felt that caring for someone with Robert's issues without medicine required more attention and work, and that the capacity and interest to do this in hospitals and care facilities was, "in reality, just not there". This left her balancing her need for support that couldn't be provided at home and her wish for Robert to get a certain type of care and to avoid medicines that might not be required. Mandy felt a profound sense of guilt that she would need to sacrifice this preference, this sense of what the best care for Robert was, to keep them both safe. In the end, for all her effort, Mandy felt that she was left with no other options and no real choices.

People with dementia and those around them often grapple with this uncertainty: are genuine choices available to them? For some people with dementia the worry is whether they have any real choice in what their future with dementia holds:

Nancy, an 83-year-old woman with moderately advanced dementia, described really wanting to "hold on" to herself to keep herself in one piece against dementia's tugging at her edges. Nancy used to be a nurse and remembered working with alcoholics and frail people in a busy metropolitan hospital in her youth. These people would "lose it" and become different and frightening. Nancy deeply hoped she wouldn't be like that, wouldn't turn into someone frightening and different. But in expressing her hope that she wouldn't become one of these lost people she also expressed some sense of equanimity in that, without the power to change this, why be upset about it? She said, "I don't mean to lose it, I really don't, but what can I do to hold it? It is not as if you can tie it up with a piece of string or something."

There is a deep wisdom here that relates to a continuing argument about how much choice any of us really has in our lives. Many contend that the array and interconnection of influences on us all means that the notion of our free will and our autonomy is just a story that we like to tell ourselves.[35] However, an important additional idea to consider is one suggested in the seventeenth century by Dutch philosopher, Baruch Spinoza. Spinoza argued that we always have choices available to us, namely, the choice of how to respond to the unavoidable realities that life presents to us (de Spinoza, 2001). In this sense (and as described so poignantly by Nancy) although we cannot tie our lives up in a piece of string and hold them as we would like them, the possibility that we can choose how we want to inhabit our own lives remains with us regardless of challenges like dementia.

But if peoples' choices are influenced by many factors, the choices of people with dementia are more so. Challenges to a person with dementia's decision-making occur on multiple levels. French psychiatrist and philosopher, Jacques Lacan, described a way of categorising the multiple levels on which these sorts of challenges can exist in his theory of three registers or interconnected and mutually dependent levels of how people experience themselves and their world: namely, the imaginary, the symbolic and the real. Let us examine these a little further and see how they clarify the decision-making challenges of people with dementia. On the imaginary level, people with dementia often imagine themselves and are perceived by others as subject to the decisions and agency of others and as having interests and wishes that are of less value and are more likely to be ignored. The people with dementia I spoke to often said that they had strong feelings about some topics but suspected that their views would not have much impact on what would occur. This was often echoed by family carers and clinicians involved in their care and their decision-making. Involving people with dementia in discussion of choices was seen as an "aggravation" and hearing (and often ignoring) their wishes a "dreary" if necessary process. Lacan's second inter-related register level is the symbolic register. This is the level where our experiences are influenced by other forces such as language and culture which reinforce the reality they describe (Žižek, 2006a). For people with dementia, it is in this register that our language and cultural assumptions lead to people with dementia being controlled by others. The clear power-imbalances within our systems for dealing with decision-making for people with cognitive impairment highlight how valid and powerful this symbolic register can be. Clinicians involved in supporting decision-making for people with dementia talked about avoiding realistic discussion of what the future might hold when asked by people with dementia but would instead offer "a positive sort of hope, rather than the future" that they really expected. These two registers, the symbolic structures that diminish the relevance of people with dementia's contribution to their decision-making, and the (imaginary) experienced reality of this occurring, can seem to lead networks to simply avoid involving people with dementia in decisions entirely, as when Ellen (the wife of Tim, a 68-year-old man with moderate dementia) explained that, when they disagreed, she'd allow his amnesia to work for her getting her way, saying, "Well, if he gets crabby, I just don't talk and go and do something else and it all goes away." While power imbalances are not intended, they are nevertheless an unavoidable result of the way that dementia and those with the diagnosis are regarded.

And yet, Lacan suggests that the experience of humanity is not limited to the imaginary and the symbolic registers but also includes a third register, "the real". This (real) aspect of our experience cannot be represented (Johnston, 1997b). For the decision-making of people with dementia, this element encompasses the frequent and contradictory way in which people with dementia exercise great power over the people and the systems on which they rely, and which decide for them. The physical dependence and communication challenges of persons with dementia in my research meant that decisions made "for" them often had the deepest impact on others. The vulnerability of persons with dementia also had its own compelling weight. Paul and Grace (whose mother had advanced dementia and very limited remaining verbal communication) talked about how strong they felt their mother was and their own feelings of weakness and grief at having decided to place her in an aged care facility. They felt that their mum's strength was such that she "thinks deep in her head [that] she might come out of there". She was seen by them as a resolute power contained within the form of a woman who was highly dependent and incredibly frail. Persons with dementia often had this powerful, motivating frailty. Alphonso Lingis describes something like this when he writes about how arresting and forceful the presence of the sick and the dying is. They force us out of our comfort zones and compel us to stop, think and evaluate (Lingis, 1994). The powerful presence and impact of people with dementia had a significant influence on family carers and health carers and compelled challenges to usual practice within healthcare systems. Despite the vulnerability and dependence of people with dementia and the systems that tend to diminish their experience of control over their decisions, they still have a fundamental impact on the networks that surround them.

The burden of choice

While people with dementia and their networks feel that decision-making is important, they also describe how taxing, burdensome and distressing it can be. Decision-making, to some degree, implies that there are valid choices available, but people with dementia and their carers didn't usually feel this was true for them. Carers described their distress at the lack of any good options to decide between, and their discomfort at still being made to choose and to be responsible for those choices and their outcomes. This created a sense of grief and impotency at being forced to be involved, resulting sometimes in a wish that someone else would just step in and take on the problem. Jenny (the wife of Ronald, an 87-year-old man who had moderate dementia) described it feeling easier and safer to avoid decisions rather than having to face up to making them. Jenny described herself as being like the figure in Munch's *The Scream* (1883) in those moments when she struggled to find someone to answer a question or was left with an impossible choice. She felt she was howling inside while needing to publicly keep it together to have some chance of moving forward. Another family member (Paul, the son of Mary who had advanced dementia) described his deep wish that the biggest decisions (such as deciding that the family could no longer care for a person with dementia safely at home) weren't left to family members. He felt that healthcare providers should have the responsibility for deciding these sorts of matters after assessing all of the options available. In effect, family members expressed a wish to be more informed and more closely involved until the point that being involved created too much uncertainty or moral distress, wishing at this point that they could hand on the responsibility to others. Interestingly, however, trained healthcare providers describe similar concerns. They felt uncomfortable at having to be involved in such difficult decisions without easy answers. Unlike family members, health carers seemed to be able to, and often did, focus their responsibilities on other things and limited their roles in decision-making. This, in effect, left family carers and people with dementia to grapple with the most impossible choices by themselves. Correspondingly, many expressed their sense that being recognised as a surrogate decision-maker was a burden, rather than a benefit. Having this role of decision-maker was generally not valued as an opportunity to act and extend a person with dementia's autonomy.

Surrogate decision-makers seemed to feel more like the slowest child in musical chairs, staring back at those who'd been quick enough to avoid being singled out. Decision-making in this situation then became a painful necessity and a reminder of the unwanted changes to lives that were occurring all around the person with dementia rather than drawing people together through the opportunity to provide support.

Decision-making in dementia takes place all the time and is important. In talking to people with dementia and their communities, it seemed that decision-making was more noteworthy and obvious than in other circumstances as it involved new considerations, unfamiliar processes and painful challenges. Decision-making was also deeply meaningful, but perhaps not always in the way we might expect. Decisions in dementia weren't just meaningful because they involved difficult choices, though difficult choices were common, but because decisions related to and expressed many things. An important aspect of this was that decision-making expressed aspects — the different selves — of the people who were involved in making them. Decisions expressed people's identities, enacted and refreshed their stories and explored what they valued. They also did this in a way which was visible and recountable: like stepping stones rising above the churning waters, decisions were remembered and shared and revealed much. Decisions were about what people felt and wanted individually and collectively, and the process of trying to work through complexity often entailed insight. Decisions also showed how difficult the challenges and changes that were frequently part of dementia were for those involved. In a way, while decisions were invariably related to how the future might be, and what could be done to make it more like a future that those involved wanted, they were also closely tied to how the present was experienced, and how people remembered their past together. This reflective process of decision-making could be seen as constructing a kind of bridge or link between these different times and parts of people affected with dementia, who they were, who they are, and who they might be.

4. Our, not your, dementia

Dementia involves and is inseparable from relationships. As we've discussed, how we relate to people with dementia shapes what "dementia" means, and this is true within our large communities and within the smaller regions of dementia networks. A key manifestation of this relationality within dementia networks relates to ideas of providing care. At some stage, when people live with dementia, care and support become a necessity. That's more broadly true of all of us, though. If you consider care as Joan Tronto and Berenice Fisher do as everything that we do to maintain, continue and repair our world (including our bodies and our selves), to live in it as well as we can, then we're all involved in giving and receiving care (Tronto, 2020). Particular types of care, though, are more common in dementia due to the physical, social and psychological dependencies associated with its cognitive and communicative frailty. People with advancing dementia need more help in many forms. That essentially means they need more people, or more of other people. As we've also noted, though, care in dementia as elsewhere is a relational practice that requires human connection and engagement. We need people to connect for care to happen. So, it is not surprising that care and relationships would seem aligned when you talk to dementia networks, or that the experience of dementia involves more than just the person with the diagnosis. In talking to people with dementia, their family carers and those involved in providing them with clinical care, it was clear that relationships are a potent force in dementia. Relationships involved change. In my study, relationships were impacted by dementia but also had an impact on dementia itself. Relationships therefore were important and filled with meaning and showed that there was a lot at stake. Relationships were also often difficult, filled with conflict and were a struggle to maintain.

Threads in the web

Dementia didn't mean that relationships lost meaning. Far from it. Relationships, particularly those between family carers and people living with dementia, involved feelings of belonging and mutual understanding which continued or even became heightened through dementia. The experience of these deep relationships seemed an ongoing central point to the worlds of those involved. Relationships also provided evidence for how people with dementia still had a place in this world (Agich, 1993b). They had a place with their family, friends and communities. They were connected to them in a "web" of connected threads, links and shared experiences. The thicker the web, replete with these sorts of links and connections, the greater the protection these relationships seemed to provide against dementia's slow but persistent erosive impact on the web's structure. Carers (particularly family members) and people with dementia talked about how they buttressed the web and rekindled their connection to each other through demonstrating their shared respect, commitment, values and history with each other. Dementia, in this sense, hadn't stopped how these people still "fit each other" and "balanced each other out". In older couples, when one person had dementia and the other (often) didn't, their relationship often included a shared sense that needing care and support was actually a familiar experience for both of them, and not unique to the person with dementia. Neither of them was getting younger and they were both "going downhill together" and the dementia was just one kind of hill. This often meant that these people felt more able to understand and appreciate what the other was going through. The need for care in these kinds of relationships could be something that drew people together rather than made them feel separate.

Relationships seemed to have a stabilising effect on the experience of dementia for people with the diagnoses, where strong connected webs were comfortable, reliable, and reassuring. Relationships were also seen as a potentially resilient part of the person with dementia's experience. Relationships had more potential give and flex than many other parts of the person with dementia's world. Changes in memory, for instance, had little give: you either had that experience or you didn't. But changes in relationships had extra supports built in. Problems and challenges could, to some extent, be accommodated and managed. This stabilising quality of relationships meant that they often became an even more important source of confidence and connection, particularly for persons with dementia, a sanctuary which was resistant to the new challenges and uncertainties that were arising. Even new relationships with people with shared experiences (such as those formed within dementia support groups) were appreciated as a source of support by people with dementia and carers. People with dementia, for instance, described such groups as being in "one channel" with each other. They were a new community whose members could understand each other and could rapidly become a new avenue of strength and support. The importance of these new relationships wasn't limited to people with a shared experience. People with dementia also described healthcare providers and care workers as "friends". This supported some people with dementia to feel cared for and that they "belonged" in environments where their new friends worked, such as aged care facilities. Connections and relationships could provide new strength and confidence for dementia networks, particularly for the people with dementia when they needed it most.

Identity and intelligibility

Relationships also cared for things besides whole people. They had a critical role in creating, maintaining and expressing identity. They reinforced and challenged how people saw themselves and each other. They contributed to a shared repository of experiences, language and memories from which identity arose. But they also provided a means to reflect on whether old identities and roles still fit and what they meant to those involved now. People with dementia and those around them identified themselves relative to others. They were who they were because of the roles they fulfilled for each other and the connections arising from these roles. Healthcare providers described having identities like being the "captain of the ship" or the "change-agent". These identities were powerful independent leaders, or flexible collaborators, and involved the freedom to choose how and when they should be involved in situations, like providing care. Healthcare providers also identified themselves relative to those they were involved in caring for in some instances. Some saw themselves as people who value others living with dementia or as "companions" supporting them during their illness journey, both identities implying a greater sense of responsibility, greater rewards and greater risks due to their deeper connection to those people living with dementia and their carers with whom they worked.

Carers expressed the understandable impact their relationships with people living with dementia had had on their own identities. They commonly voiced their uncertainty at whether they were "a carer now" instead of, or in addition to, the other things that they'd previously been in relation to the person with dementia — like a friend, a lover, a partner or a child. They had often noticed a particular change in how they were with the person living with dementia, too — their time with the person living with dementia now seemed primarily focused on monitoring and supporting them. The times when their life together had been about supporting and being with each other often seemed to have passed. For some, the new and unfamiliar intimacies and vulnerabilities associated with this new "carer" role created challenges due to unfamiliarity and inexperience, and feelings that being involved in this kind of moment was inappropriate. Others experienced these awkward and uncertain vulnerabilities as something that reinforced their sense of their relationships with those around them. People living with dementia and carers described feeling something that was kindled within their roles of family-member, spouses or friends for each other. Stories, moments of humour, shared memories and touch played an increasingly important role in appreciating connections. Mike (son of Nellie, an 86-year-old woman with advanced dementia) shared a story of taking Nellie to the dentist, which involved them negotiating a significant and worrying climb up a large flight of stairs to get to the office. There were risky moments involved but Mike's recollection was one of wistful fondness and humour:

> "I said, 'There you go mum, you have made it to Mount Everest' and she said, 'feels like it'. [strong laughter] … She is really on the ball at times and comes out with stuff like that and your heart just melts. That is my mum [cries quietly]."

In these shared moments, it was clear that the person living with dementia was "still there", allowing their identity and the related identities of others to feel resonant and secure. People living with dementia also expressed the importance of their past roles to who they felt they were now. While the roles themselves (such as jobs, or community or professional appointments) were often now inactive, the relationships associated with these, with colleagues and friends, were active and empowering. All manner of relationships, not just close relationships between people who saw each other often and had closely intertwined lives, were potentially important contributors to how people living with dementia and those around them saw themselves and each other.

How well identities continued to work within relationships, how well the identity continued to fit or continued to seem intelligible within that relationship was a common trigger of new challenges. Relationships and the people within them felt intelligible if their identities cohered with pre-existing and assumed structures within that network of people. For instance, changing roles associated with a need to provide or receive more physical care felt inconsistent with role assumptions for many people, making understanding those roles and the identities behind them more difficult. A common example was when those who were the children of people living with dementia were in situations where they needed to start providing physical care for their parents who had dementia. Needing to help a parent use the toilet is challenging for many reasons, with one being that the role and identity of "parent" is associated with giving support to vulnerable family members rather than having to receive it. Describing a "parent" as someone who only provides care is clearly a simplification but, still, the role includes all sorts of unsaid but powerful assumptions. Children in this situation often expressed this as a kind of unnatural discomfort, an upturning of what their parent was for them due to this new facet to their roles for each other. Those carers in effect wondered what "parent" means and whether this term changes over time from someone who is a support to someone who requires support from others. Social structures (such as schools and healthcare institutions) anticipate norms and normalise relationships in ways which formalise and solidify the power differences within our society (Foucault, 2012). This is even true of families, where the roles we live and set for ourselves and each other, while undergoing constant cultural shifts, determine what sort of behaviour makes sense (C. Taylor, 2012). When people conform to the norms which are expected within and by social structures, they are intelligible to their community, they fit and make sense within their community. Being a parent and care-recipient might not make sense based on some norms of what these roles mean but that wasn't true for everyone. Some children seemed to feel that the parent-child role was more about reciprocity and giving back rather than care needing to move in one direction. For those people, it seemed easier to fit the idea of having a parent with dementia who also required their physical care within their sense of their world.

What makes a role intelligible is sometimes clear. In dementia networks, healthcare providers had roles which were understood as having certain types of power relative to other network members. Exercising these powers (such as making a diagnosis or recommending an approach to responding to a problem) was expected and doing so made the person and the role make sense to everyone because they were fulfilling what was expected of them. Within families and friends of people with dementia, role expectations were more reliant on those involved in these relationships to decide together what still worked and whether identities made sense. This reciprocal discovery that roles continued to make sense could be incredibly important to people with dementia and carers. June (a 73-year-old woman with mild dementia) talked about how discussions with her son (Roy) had supported them both in feeling they were doing as well as they could, given the situation. June shared a situation when Roy had told her that his ability to cope and be flexible was his "taking after his mum", highlighting how their shared commitment to loving and supporting each other made their situation more bearable — because they were in it together. Their roles for each other as son and mother had changed but still made sense to them within this context of shared respect and love.

Dementia could also make the expression of identity much less clear, and relationships often came to the rescue. For example, carers often had such clear knowledge of the person with dementia and a familiarity with how their communication had changed that they spoke for this person. By this I mean that they helped clarify and amplify what the person with dementia was trying to communicate in a way which made their views much easier to understand. In the examples I'm thinking of this was being done with the person with dementia present and agreeing with what the carer suggested, and so these moments seemed like the family was interpreting the world for the person with dementia, and the person with dementia for the world. These relationships, therefore, made the views of people with dementia more accessible and apparent. Their identity would be much more clearly seen and would be informed by the person with dementia. These relationships also simultaneously provided carers with the authority and proximity to validly speak on the person with dementia's behalf and for this to be accepted and compelling. Relationships helped determine whether people with dementia remained intelligible within the network and, in doing so, created this reality (Foucault, 1978).

Network members in different roles and relationships had different expectations regarding what was intelligible for them. For many family carers, the inter-mixing of expected norms involved in being both a carer and a family member required constant work to remain intelligible. Mandy (wife of Robert, an 82-year-old with advanced dementia) spoke about becoming a "blurter" in trying to achieve this balance: "I blurt things out very quickly now because if I am on the phone I might have to get off at any minute. So, I blurt things out in a rush and tell everybody everything." There simply wasn't enough time to hold all of her relationships and roles. For Mandy, the only way to keep her connections and maintain her other roles was to accept that her role as carer had to be the priority and could tear her away from others at any time. Success in remaining intelligible in these roles required the prioritisation of contrasting goals such as dedication, self-care, and altruism. The tipping point between what's best care for the person with dementia and what's best for the carer was frequently a difficult balance to maintain. While some people felt that this was indeed a balance that they had managed to maintain, it was often a process that was painful and destructive. However, when this balance wasn't maintained, a new slew of different relationship, identity and role challenges could arise — as a sustained imbalance often led to questions of admission to hospital or placement of the person with dementia in some sort of care facility.

Identities, by and large, seemed to be more likely to still fit and work if everything else (such as the relationships within the network) all seemed to be staying the same. This might have been why people living with dementia tended to interpret and describe their relationships with carers (particularly those with close family and partners) as unchanged, even while changes were clearly continuing. The logic here is that if, say, I'm in an unchanged relationship with my wife, then a whole bunch of other statuses and identities, like being best-friends, lovers, parents, home-owners, etc., all seem fairly solid. On the other hand, if our relationship changed significantly then at least some of these other things might too, and we'd be different people for each other and may feel like different people ourselves. For some persons living with dementia their sense that their connections to others weren't changed meant they could also see themselves as the same as they'd always been. They still knew themselves and described themselves as professionals, respected members of their community, and as treasured partners and family members. These identities and roles made sense because they seemed to be supported by relationships which made them make sense, and all of this was a webbing to support the person to remain stably within their network. Carers also had an active role in helping out with similar processes. How they described their relationships did however seem influenced by whether the person with dementia was involved in the conversation, as carers were often less confident about relationships remaining unchanged in private with me. Carers also noted their attempts to maintain the social identity of the persons with dementia by supporting what they used to do for them. This could be through helping them in unacknowledged ways to attend gatherings or fulfil social obligations. Carers were therefore working hard with people with dementia to support them to feel nothing had changed — and working hard around the person with dementia to support everyone else to feel that nothing had changed. Doing this with any success did, somewhat ironically, lead to changing identity. It led to the carer being identified as a skilled care provider and a good or loving family member or partner. In some situations, doing all of this actually mattered more for the carer than the person with dementia. People with more advanced dementia seemed to care less about these identities, but carers enabling that identity to continue supported networks in being able to see a treasured part of the person with dementia be maintained for as long as possible.

Power and the person

As Michel Foucault observed, "where there is power, there is resistance", and the paradoxical co-relationship of these factors can be seen in the workings of dementia networks (Foucault, 1978). All members of the network seemed to have the ability to influence and to create resistance. Interestingly, at least a share of the resistance in the networks seemed to be that of network members trying to avoid having influence and power over what was to happen to the person with dementia. Carers and health carers clearly both had power and influence in networks and generally acknowledged this. Health carers were empowered by their roles within the network. Health carers had access to skills, activities and interventions of various types due to these being afforded to them by the healthcare system. However, while health carers were happy to exercise the powers specifically within their role, they tended to resist having a broader power in influencing the network. Sometimes health carers didn't seem to know or respect the potency and impact of their words and their roles. Beatrice (77-year-old with mild dementia) shared a story about how disempowered she was by the well-intentioned actions of her doctor:

> Beatrice had been working in an office for many years when her dementia was diagnosed. It was difficult to get the diagnosis. She

had mild dementia and needed to see a number of specialists prior to getting the answer. She'd had a conversation with her GP after the news came back and they'd talked about how her work was getting more difficult. They'd planned to keep talking about that and Beatrice thought nothing of it. What she didn't realise though was that her doctor felt that the right thing to do was to write to her workplace to see whether her work could become more flexible, given her diagnosis. The doctor's heart was in the right place but her head was somewhere else, Beatrice thought. The doctor never asked her whether they should do that and if she had done so Beatrice would have told her, "That was the worst thing she could have done." Within a week of receiving the letter, Beatrice said, "(her boss) had (her) put off on a pension."

The carers of people with dementia often did not want the power they felt they had, but also did not feel that they had the power to rescind it. Carers, by virtue of their role, were on the one hand empowered because they cared for someone who was dependent on that care. But that connection cut two ways, and they were also at the mercy of this care responsibility with little opportunity (unlike health carers) to say, "That's someone else's job to sort out". Family carers felt their lives were overrun by the responsibility to provide care. They also felt that these challenges and requirements for care were not understood by others, that they "don't get it", meaning that they also had to spend a lot of time defending and explaining why their days were so challenging. This was a huge weight for many to carry and many were struck by being unable to stop being a carer, even when it was their preference to do so. Even for those who felt that they had been able to walk away from their role, the personal costs seemed high. Joan (daughter of Nellie an 86-year-old with advanced dementia) described her response to placing her mum in an aged care facility when she could no longer care for her safely at home:

> "I had flung her back into this institution and just bolted, just gone … It's what I did to my mum. It's what I did to my mum, I chucked her in there."

Even with the apparent power to be able to make decisions and to remove themselves from roles, family carers felt far from powerful and sometimes seemed powerless to carry on with what they felt they had had to do. The risk of "losing track" of the person with dementia (and them losing track of their family) when "you hand them over" to other people to look after them was seen as a huge risk that might result from being less involved, particularly if that resulted in admission to an aged care facility. All participants largely lacked the power to self-determine their status within their relationships with other network members due to the complexity of interconnections between them. This was most true for persons with dementia. People with dementia often felt misunderstood and under-appreciated by those around them but felt that they had limited chance to correct the ledger, and few alternative choices. Carers could (at least in principle) walk away from their care roles and determine their own boundaries and limits, while persons with dementia were highly dependent on their network and the relationships that formed it.

• • •

Power and resistance also seemed key contributors to the process of discovering identity. Foucault suggested that it is through being subject to structures of power, and through our own response to them that we are "attached" to our own identity (Foucault, 1982). Such attachment to identities which were central to the interplay of power and its resistance were frequent for people in dementia networks. The "extra duties" that family carers now felt they had responsibility for colonised all the available space, challenging and subsuming every other part of their relationships with the person with dementia. It was common for carers to describe feeling as though "being a carer now" was suffocating all of the other identities that they'd had for and with the person with dementia. Trying to focus on what was left of their pre-carer relationships with the person with dementia was an act of resistance. This could be through making sure that, when new people came into the picture, they knew that there was more to the relationship than just being "carer" and the "person who receives care", or by prioritising activities that were reminders of how the relationship had once been — acts against the dominance of the carer role and reminders of what had been lost. Carers also sought to find extra meaning, beyond just providing care, within the role (in part to sustain themselves). Caring can partly become grieving, as losses of relationships and of parts of the person with dementia become more and more difficult to cover over

(Hennings et al., 2010). In my study, these difficulties were exacerbated for carers by being placed in what were felt to be relationally or culturally "unnatural" situations, such as carers who'd previously been a more submissive partner now making the decisions, negotiating bathing for proud and dignified family members, or children providing personal care for their parents. Throughout, carers also needed to strike a balance between the needs of the person with dementia and their own needs. They were left in a "limbo land" of understanding the expectations of those around them but being unable to meet or reconcile them.

Change

While relationships adhered people in dementia networks to each other and their world, they were not static. The changing nature of relationships within the dementia network was a core element of their experience of dementia. Change in relationships over time affected how relationships were understood and what they meant. But the interpretation of relationships and their changes was not uniform. Different members of the network experienced and interpreted what was occurring and what it meant in different ways. Changes in relationships were difficult, and difficult to discuss. People commonly expressed their ongoing love, respect, commitment and reliance, but these experiences didn't mean that there weren't also difficulties and pressures associated with relationship changes. Honestly, I think it's likely that even in the best of times it's difficult to talk to someone else about how your relationship is changing. But, talking to a partner that you've had for 50 years and who now also has cognitive and communicative changes, or a parent who knows their memory is unreliable but is desperate to cover for it because they don't want to be sent to a home, about what you feel is difficult for you now, is not the best of times. The frustrations of trying to find the right time and manner to talk about what had changed and for this to feel safe and understood meant that this was an easy topic to avoid discussing. An open discussion of change sometimes made clear the disempowerment that people with dementia felt. They often now felt an expectation to be passive, voiceless recipients of the actions of others.

Changing relationships had changing dynamics. People with dementia were frequently side-lined because the primary person in the relationship who shared what had happened to them and what things meant was someone else who "hadn't forgotten" as they were prone to do. More subtle still was the changing intent behind relationships that seemed superficially similar, such as people with dementia's connections to workplaces and professional groups, when people with dementia were allowed to continue to "be a part of it to make (them) feel that (they) are still in the loop". These kinds of relationships seemed a consolation and an act of generosity or pity, rather than a genuine, mutual connection. Relationship changes could be isolating for family carers as they often felt that they were the only one who was bereaved, due to the person with dementia not seeming to mourn changes in relationships in the same way. Jenny (wife of Ronald, an 84-year-old man with moderate dementia) described changes to conversation:

> "We used to talk for a long time about what had happened during the day ... but that doesn't happen at all now ... no there's not what I would call a conversation at all now. I don't suppose Ronald misses it, but I do."

Family carers felt unsure how they could grieve the changes that were occurring while maintaining and developing a relationship with the person they were caring for. Graham (partner of Darren a 64-year-old with mild dementia) talked about how Darren's dementia seemed to speed up the deteriorating links of the "cobweb" of connections around them:

> "... in the end you end up with all these little separate parts of the cobweb but they are not connected anymore ... you are on your little island. They are on their little island."

Losing connection to others, to the person with dementia, even to health carers as needs changed and ending up on a cluster of little islands seemed a common risk.

• • •

Despite all of this, changes in relationships did not always denote loss. New relationships arose and grew out of the field of the dementia experience. Some new relationships, such as those between people with dementia, were objects of wonder. In these new relationships, carers and health carers commented that people with dementia could be speaking "their own language", seemingly meaningless or at the least inaccessible to those people without dementia but clearly creating a "human connection" which was readily understood by everyone. Regardless, the content of that connection and what it meant remained private and available only to the people with dementia involved. Carers in particular expressed their mixed responses to changes in relationships. While unwanted changes were distressing and a source of grief, there were also more positive changes, sometimes fleeting or incomplete, but these were sources of joy and comfort.

Levels of meaning

The meanings of our relationships, connections, roles and identities and what influences how these grow and shape is complex terrain. An important point here is that the connections between people aren't just influenced by those people involved. A host of other things play into what happens — including our language, culture and our shared (or contested) sense of what things mean. We'll return to this idea later in the book, but for now let's think through what the dementia networks we heard from seem to suggest about the different processes that affect roles and relationships at play. To try and break these processes down into a structure we'll again use Lacan's registers.[36] As we've discussed, these registers, what he called the symbolic, the imaginary and the real (Johnston, 1997a), are a way of seeing human experience and interconnection and are interlinked and co-dependent. For Lacan the imaginary represents how we interpret our world around us and how our relationship to our interpretation affects and compels us; the symbolic is the unconscious organisation of human society including how that is manifest in language, law and social structures; and the real is the indescribable, and unsymbolised "the thing in itself" elements of our experience (Bailly, 2009; Ribolsi et al., 2015; Žižek, 2006a). Using this structure, we can work through the impact of dementia on relationships within that network of people. On an imaginary level, aspects of the experience of relationships were being re-interpreted by people in the network, while the symbolic status of network members including the language used to describe them and what society felt that they should or must do was also changing. Family carers who were grieving their "losing track" of persons with dementia on an imaginary level were also, on a symbolical level, failing to perform as carers and as loved ones within the crucible of dementia's challenge. Persons with dementia experienced changes to their connection with others and in the meaning of those changes on an imaginary level, while also feeling that they were symbolically branded by the dementia, its effects and others' expectations. This branding was deep and pervasive. The interests, preferences and experiences of persons with dementia were liable to being symbolically devalued as uninterpretable (for instance by being actively or passively excluded from their own decision-making), even as their views were determined as highly precious within the imaginary sphere, expressing something fundamental about who they continued to be.

Culture and language made important contributions to the symbolic interpretation of relationships. Much of this contribution is entrenched and inconspicuous. Caring roles are gendered due to historical, cultural and linguistic conventions (Haraway, 2015; Irigaray, 1985). The cost of caring and how that impacts on those, mostly women, who provide care is often hidden and the work of caring is considered as a normal thing for women (rather than men) in society to provide (Morgan et al., 2016). Carers in this study were often women and their ongoing contribution to care was seen as necessary, required and appropriate, adhering to common (symbolic) beliefs around the performance of these sorts of roles (Williams et al., 2017). Adequately performing these caring norms, particularly for family carers of people with dementia required the, often undiscussed, adoption of this dominant and overwhelming role while also keeping it partially hidden and in balance with other things.

The finding that dementia care is culturally and socially assumed as being women's work is not that surprising. However, focusing on this a little further might help us in thinking through and describing some of the challenges that dementia network members face. We're going to do that by using some of the work of Donna Haraway, an influential feminist thinker. In a famous essay from 1985, Haraway described her sense that women in particular (and people more generally) were in a flux of conflicting states of wholeness and fragmentation being driven by a host of different tensions within culture and language, contested statuses, and levels of meaning which overlap, co-exist and remain unresolved. Haraway suggested that this meant we should see and understand them not as a single, defined, solitary something but more like an amalgam of meanings, a cluster of potentially contradictory ideas within our chaotic, constructed world. Haraway's suggestion was that rather than a woman (or person) being defined as a single thing we

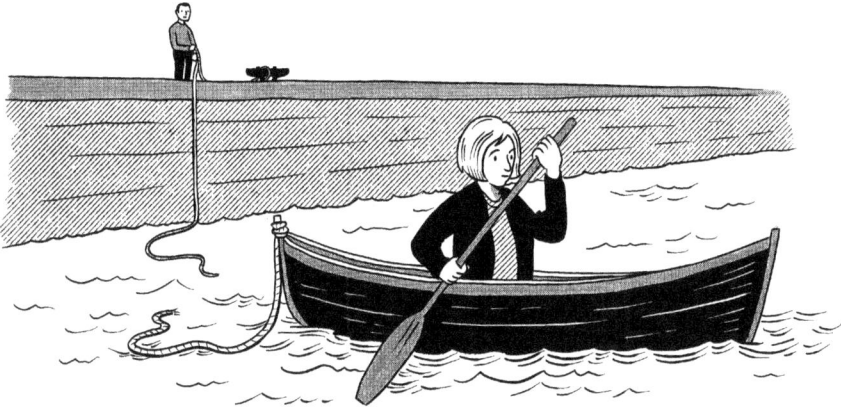

could instead consider them as a "cyborg" (or cybernetic organism) —
existing within a continuum of tensions between human and animal,
human and machine, the material and the immaterial (Haraway, 1991).
The cyborg idea was a way of trying to grasp this complex idea that a
person can be fragmented and dispersed while also being quite clearly
apparent, solid and real.

We can use this idea of the cyborg as a tool to provide some
extra language and analysis of the challenges faced by people within
dementia networks. Extending this idea to the family carers of people
with dementia (who were often women), they were cyborgs in their
simultaneous and un-relenting requirement to be a loved/loving
person and a carer, to have roles to support and to compel, and to
flex to the needs of others while being and seeming to be unchanged
and unchallenged. The notion of the cyborg may also be helpful in
considering the impact of dementia on people living with the diagnosis.
As we've discussed, persons with dementia are fragmented, and
symbolically scattered. When thinking about a person with dementia
we might be thinking about the stigma of their illness, our terror of
meeting a similar fate, about how they act as a purposeless reminder
of loss, how they represent a major social and healthcare problem, and
about them as an unchanged person despite their condition. Rather
than seeking to resolve these singular expectations it may be that the
best way to understand the experience of a family carer or person with
dementia is to view them as such a cyborg, emerging from the multiple
tensions that confront them. For people with dementia this might
include us suggesting that the dementia experience simultaneously
and conflictingly includes: the individual with dementia as a being,

and their dementia as a monstrous or animal descent; the demarcation between the natural frailty of the human and the assisted persistence of the person; and the bodily and impactful presence of the person with dementia along with the uncertainty of their participation in shifting the world around them. In symbolically allowing the person with dementia to exist across complexities and tensions (similar to those who care for them) we provide room for the dynamic and complex experiences that occur between the unique and enmeshed people that make up their networks. This position also suggests a symbolic recognition of an experience that defies clear external definition. It allows the person with dementia to be understood as speaking "their own language" with a real experience that is beyond the imaginary understanding of others.

Relationships between network members also occurred on deeper levels that cannot be clearly defined. They often did not rely on language but occurred through the bare simplicity of the connection with the other. For Lacan this could be considered a connection that occurs through a real register of experience, an experience that is fundamental and unaffected by interpretation. This "real" level or register seems unknowable but feels tied to the deep, immediate, human bodily need of people with dementia and their networks to value and to be valued, to care and be cared for underlying the sometimes-overwhelming changes to experience and relationships that are occurring. Family carers described the importance of pure physical connection as contributing to the meaning of their relationship. This embodied relational connection does not necess-arily require touch, but a connection associated with being together. Levinas describes such levels of connection as pre-conceptual and pre-linguistic (Levinas, 1981). It is in the movement towards the other demanded by the challenge of their presence (their face) that this connection happens. Such connection can and does occur without language and forms the basis of all relationships, including those involving persons with dementia's significant communicative changes. While clearly instrumental in family carers' understanding of their ongoing connection to persons with dementia, the immediacy of the connection to the "face" of the person with dementia also has relevance to relationships with health carers. The initial seed of the need to care, and to notice, or the discomfort at not feeling we can achieve this lies within the "face" of the person with dementia.

Our dementia

In my study, relationships within dementia networks were complex, changing, meaningful and a significant influence on how dementia was experienced. They influenced how participants saw and understood themselves, and others. They were affected by the differences in power between individual participants, which was also influenced by cultural, linguistic and community expectations of how such interactions should occur. As a result, systems of meaning developed within and around the dementia network affecting the experience of ongoing connection between its members. While persons with dementia were considered dependent, they were also the centre of the care network, and powerful contributors to their relationships with others. The importance of relationships in creating and maintaining experience, identity, connection, narrative and the symbolic importance of roles and responsibilities means that dementia is something that "we" experience rather than a problem for individuals.

This notion, that dementia is something that is experienced by people, rather than by a single person with a diagnosis, has clearly been evident from the results of speaking to people with dementia and their networks which has been the basis for this chapter. Our initial discussion of the "dementia manifold" showed us that the dementia experience includes not only a variety of ongoing changes but the expectation of what those changes can and will mean, and what responses are available to them. This was a continual process, not halted by the progression of dementia and the loss of communication, that involved many people seeking to make sense of the unfolding of what was occurring. Similarly, decision-making conceived as "stepping stones" influencing the path of the river of dementia represented how decisions are a complicated business in dementia. Multiple people are involved and manifold different meanings are likely from the process and the results, with the stakes being the possibility of coherence (through decision-making) of who those people affected by dementia were, are and who they will be.

While not an exhaustive or universal account of all that can be learned from talking to people with dementia and those closest to them this central message, that dementia is not a simple condition in an individual person, is clear. Dementia is not a single diagnosis, a simple change in memory, or a cognitive test score. It doesn't have a solitary meaning, a uniform future or completely predictable parts.

Dementia is not "hopeless", and it is not a liberation. But all of these ideas come from somewhere. To some extent, while dementia is none of these things, it is also clearly all of these things to some people some of the time. Dementia involves many ideas and many interpretations from many people. It has levels of meaning and interpretation and the results are more the accumulation or assemblage of tensions or contradictions than they resolve away into a simple answer.

In short, dementia is complex and involves a lot of interconnected parts. While that might seem too brief a summary, this notion of the complexity of interconnections within what we call dementia is central to what we'll discuss from here in our efforts to try to understand the experience of dementia more than we currently do.

PART THREE

From networks to systems

Part Three proposes a different way to think about dementia networks and the experience of dementia through understanding them as living systems. In Chapter One ("Systems and complexity"), I explain in theoretical terms what I mean by systems, how this relates to people's communication, how people see themselves and how they're seen by others. Chapter Two ("Systems in dementia") will start to explore what all of this means within dementia and how it applies to dementia networks. Chapter Three ("Mapping change in dementia networks") will then use these ideas to look at stories from dementia networks to try to understand what seems to be going on in those networks. This chapter liberally uses theory and ideas from the first two. Anyone experiencing some theory-fatigue, however, could skip straight to this chapter. I've re-defined key words and ideas there, but the first two chapters will still be there waiting to help out if you end up reconsidering. Chapter Four ("Making sense of change") brings this part of the book together in reviewing what changes in dementia systems look like and what they mean.

1. Systems and complexity

Dementia is not a single thing experienced by a single person. The impact of dementia ripples outwards. But the movements of the ripples, their intersections and reflections, aren't simple to predict or to chart. After the stone hits the water the ripples encounter obstructions, are enhanced by other currents and flows and they impact and are impacted by other living things that make their home there. Dementia is a complex experience which involves many people and multiple factors — such as our cultural and social beliefs regarding dementia, the language that we have available to describe it and its changes, and structures such as the law, medicine, and care services that respond to the challenges that dementia often creates.

While that might all be true, it hardly seems helpful when dementia already appeared complicated enough when we were worrying about it as a microscopic change in the brains of an increasing number of people. "How useful are these new ideas?" you could be excused for asking, if they don't actually help us respond to dementia in any kind of positive way? Well, I'm glad you asked, as this is exactly what this chapter is about.

Fortunately, a body of thinking called systems theory provides a way of conceptualising these sorts of interconnections and responses. From this perspective, dementia is not a single, specific thing, but a type of change that affects the many systems from which our living experience emerges. This is a powerful idea. Considering the problems that dementia causes us from the perspective of systems thinking enables us to confront them in new ways. It can start to help us provide some reason for why (as we've mentioned earlier) dementia affects people *and* people affect dementia. In the sections that follow we'll begin to explore what systems thinking is, where the idea has come from and what it might mean for important things that seem at stake in dementia: like our identity, our connection to others and our decision-making. We'll also begin to work through what it might mean to use systems thinking to understand and relate to dementia networks and people with dementia, and for how it might be possible to help them.

What do we mean by systems?

Systems can be and can involve many things. In systems theory, systems are considered as "a set of things — people, cells, molecules or whatever — interconnected in such a way that they produce their own pattern of behaviour over time" (Meadows, 2008). A system is not just an amount of something. It is not just piles or clumps of things. For instance, the jumble of loose Lego left out by my son in the middle of the hallway is not a system. Systems have elements, interconnections and functions or purposes through time. The life within a small tidal pool is a system, the workings of a major transnational corporation is a system, the shifting semi-predictability of the weather is a system, and the nuanced development and change of a language is a system. Systems are structures involving many connected parts that respond to everything that they are exposed to in ways that are characteristic of that system. In this sense, systems cause their own behaviour, and the ability to do this is an important part of what makes them systems (Meadows, 2008). Systemic responses are not a rational process of deciding. The elements of life in a tidal pool won't debate what should happen next if the water dries up. But the system will respond. It will change, perhaps resulting in a pool with fewer, hardier creatures, or not containing creatures visible to the human eye at all. The changes that occur will also utilise the possible responses that a system of that type can make, that is, systems will use what they've got when they respond to what's happening. Some responses reflect the relative simplicity of the system. The physical system of a car, for instance, will tend to speed up under the influence of a change like being fed more petrol. More complex systems tend to involve more elements and react in ways which are more difficult to predict. While adding more petrol to a car might have predictable results, anticipating what will happen when you add different kinds of fuel to a more complex system, like social media, is a more challenging task.

Systems are everywhere. They serve as the foundation, the weave and the interconnection of life as we know it. Systems are critical, though often under-appreciated, contributors to our human experience. A quick examination reveals that what we consider as "me" involves all kinds of systems, from the obviously apparent — my musculoskeletal system providing me with mobility — to the perceived — my system of wakefulness allowing me to be alert or asleep at regular intervals — or the un-appreciable — the system of immune cells contributing to the constant policing of what they find that they consider "me" and destroying or imprisoning everything they think is not. These systems are all human systems related to me as a solid, physical human being. Not all systems are physical, however. Moving outwards from this (admittedly already complex) start we can gain some appreciation that these systems engage with (or respond to) other systems: systems of language enabling me to communicate with other mobile, communicative systemic beings, systems of ideas and meaning, systems of signs and symbols, systems of culture, systems of religion, and systems of ethics and morality to name just a few. When you start to get down to it, so much of what we experience, what we are and what we do is the topmost visible tip of a huge and unnoticed systems iceberg.

If we accept that we participate in (and are composed of) many systems, then it seems relevant to know more about systems theory. Importantly, systems theory isn't a dismissal of our lives or our choices; it doesn't seek to refute or diminish our human experience. It is also not seeking to say that there is nothing other than systems. It is fair to say, however, that there is a lot more of our experience that does arise from systems in some way than we have likely given credit to. Systems theory itself is not an attempt to simplify, or unify, the complexity of these systems or ideas, but endeavours to explain how all of these interdependencies interrelate (Gershon, 2005). It tries to understand why things work the way that they do, and to help us have a better chance of working well with systems in a way where we can be more confident of the outcomes. Systems thinking is a term used to encapsulate the perspectives and vocabulary of ideas that can be used to understand and work with the systems that systems theory allows us to appreciate (D. H. Kim, 1999).[37]

Now to the task ahead. We've explored how the experience of dementia arises from people, not just from a single person with a diagnosis. So, in thinking through the relevance of systems thinking to dementia, let's start by examining what these ideas mean for understanding groups of people. A network of people is a special type of system, usually called a social system. Social systems are things that arise from the communication and connection of people (Luhmann, 2014b). As people interact and communicate, social systems are formed and perpetuate themselves. However, it is important to remember that the social system is not made up of a collection of "whole persons". As we've discussed, the whole person of me, Michael Chapman, is made up of many systems which interact and influence each other. Michael Chapman's immune system (for instance) may play a key and influential role in affecting how easily his neuromuscular systems can enable him to go and get himself a cup of tea. His immune system may attack nerves and muscles or his mobility may take him into an environment which impacts his immune system through exposure to COVID. As part of Michael Chapman, these systems can have a huge impact on each other and yet they are not the same system. An immune system can't ride a bicycle and a neuromuscular system can't fight an infection; they're just closely connected systems with a multitude of potential ways to influence each other. You may need an immune system to continue to have a neuromuscular system, they may function as necessary conditions for each to carry out their work, but this doesn't mean that they are the same system.[38]

Returning to social systems, German sociologist, Niklas Luhmann, argued that people give rise to the communication that makes up social systems, but it is not they who communicate. Rather, communication communicates (Luhmann, 1992). Put another way, communication is part of what the group of systems and other elements that we call a human can do, but communication doesn't involve the whole of the person at the same time, it isn't "the person" who's communicating. For example, a customer who's finished eating approaches a waiter ready to finalise her bill at the counter when both people simultaneously receive phone calls (Moeller, 2005). Each person in this instance is communicating verbally on the phone to different social systems and is communicating through their actions within a different, economic social system that involves giving and receiving payment for services. In all, multiple different systems are being simultaneously engaged and communicated with by the words and actions of these two people. Communication can't be tied to a whole person as, if that were the case, we could never participate in different communicative systems at the same time. For each system it is the communication, rather than "the person" that is central. This example also reminds us that communication includes but is not limited to speech, and that valid communication for a system is what the system finds meaningful. A vote is a valid communication for a political system, a gesture may be a valid communication for an interpersonal interaction, and stocks for a financial one. What makes these communications valid is that the system recognises and responds to them, and so it is the system which determines what valid communication means to it (D. Lee, 2000).

Inside and outside a system

Understanding living systems requires us to recognise that there are things that "are" and "are not" part of the system. In some simple systems, like the example of the car above, it's easy to determine the flow of things going into and coming out of the system: I put fuel in the car, turn it on, apply pressure to the accelerator and the system outputs movement. Living systems are a little different in that there is a separation between the system and the environment, allowing the system to develop its own responses to whatever seems to be happening. Key insights in understanding living systems arose from cellular biology, and cells are also useful in illustrating core systems principles. Cells are separated from their environment by a cellular membrane that differentiates the cell from its world. However, this membrane also connects the cell to its world. Cells and other systems are both separated from and attached to the world through their boundaries and it is through these boundaries that they interact with all that is beyond them (Boulding & Khalil, 2002).

These concepts are also relevant to social systems. Social systems also possess a dynamic boundary which both closes them off and connects them to other things allowing them to respond to influences or "perturbations" that arise from their surrounding environments. A cell or a social system determines its own response to what it encounters and engages with. You can find a dramatic example of this idea in the television drama *Severance*. In *Severance*, a group of workers has agreed to a neurological procedure. The effects of the procedure are that when they are at work in a secure, underground office, they have no memory of, or connection with, the world outside. They do have lives outside of work and yet they arrive each day at work remembering only what they've done at work with each other, and nothing else. Eventually, messages from outside get through to the group and, as an operationally closed social system which functionally only includes themselves and the barrier separating them from everything else, they need to make sense of what those messages mean to them and how they will respond. In systems theory the word for this is "autopoiesis", a capacity for self-determined change within systems, an idea which Luhmann borrowed from the work of biologists, Maturana and Varella, on other living systems (H. Maturana & Varela, 1980).

While systems are separated from their environments, much of their environment actually consists of other systems. Some of these external systems may be required for the system to function. A social system's environment includes other functionally necessary systems, such as the human biological and the psychic (or mental) systems of the persons involved within the social system (Luhmann, 2014b). For instance, for my communication to you within the social system of health literature a number of other systems are absolutely required. I need to be able to form these ideas within my mind and type them using my fingers for that communication to even begin. The systems governing my thoughts and my movements are required for this communication to be possible. This is critical for our experience as human beings. It is due to closed but connected boundaries that our mind (our psychic system) can perceive our cognitive and emotional responses and make meaning from symbols of language as we participate in the social system of communication with those around us (Moeller, 2005). Luhmann described this as "structural coupling", where systems and environments depend on the connection with each other to be able to function (Luhmann, 2014b). The various systems which contribute to making me (and you) are structurally coupled together, just as they are connected and dependent on all manner of other systems within our experienced world. What we experience as our lives is, therefore, the results of all these interlinked and mutually dependent systems of meaning, communication and physicality that are constantly influencing each other.

Systems of who we are

So far so good, but we need to go further. Systems thinking has clear if complex implications for understanding experiences of how people relate and function together. In particular, systems thinking can help us understand important experiences like our sense of identity, relationships and decision-making. These are generally formative experiences for people as well as having additional layers of importance within the experience of dementia — as we've seen in the preceding chapters. In this section, we'll explore some of the more general implications of systems thinking for identity, relationships and decision-making before considering in more detail (in "Mapping Change in Dementia Systems") how this might impact the dementia experience.

The focus on interconnectedness in systems thinking suggests that there might be value in exploring how identity, relationships and decision-making influence and relate to each other. Identity, for instance, is as we've discussed an idea that's commonly used and deeply contested. We all identify ourselves and others in ways which seem relatively stable and predictable. We've previously discussed that perhaps because I continue to experience an ongoing sense of myself (selfhood) there is an impression that the identity or identities around me are somewhat static or continuous. Considering what we've uncovered from systems thinking (not to mention from Jacques Lacan, Donna Haraway and our dementia networks) we'd have to note that identity probably isn't one thing (due to its reliance on multiple different interacting systems) and probably can't be static for similar reasons. Systems are in the business of receiving and responding to change — often to try and maintain some sort of equilibrium, but still doing so through continual change. A system no longer changing probably means that it is no longer a system. To return to thinking about identity, some of this will probably seem obvious. My identity needs to be attached to all the changing physical and mental processes involved in being me. It doesn't stop there, though. Some identities like my being a researcher, depend on a lot of additional structures beyond me (like our societies' ideas about what research is and who's allowed to do it) to make sense. Systems within me and systems outside me all play a part. So, identity arises through the experience of the interaction of our constantly changing personal (mental, physical, psychological), social and broader systems of meaning and practice.

Even if this might make some logical sense, it is difficult to avoid the assumption that we are simply ourselves. We continue to believe in an independent single self and therefore create one to fulfil this requirement. Anthropologist Gregory Bateson felt that people solidify a "self" from one (small) part of all that they are, ignoring the surrounding field of interlocking processes that get in the way of that appreciation (Bateson, 1972b). We also get a lot of help in coming to these conclusions as our perception and judgement of who we are is itself influenced by culture and language which not only support these ideas but hold up the "self-made" person as being a valuable and heroic ideal. Dementia can affect the process of a person exploring and defending their sense of their own identity (as we've suggested previously), but it may have less impact on our actual identity and where it comes from.

Let's start working through a systems' view of understanding a person with an identity. We'll start with the idea that the identity of a person is a singular thing, unique to us, which is somewhat fixed or stable. Systems theory suggests that identity is an ongoing and unending process. Seeking our identity is akin to "squaring a circle", an iterative, incremental process of constant refining (Bauman, 2004a).[39] Deleuze and Guattari suggested something similar when they talked about an individual as a "becoming": each of us is a growing, shifting process that adapts and branches in response to the world (Deleuze et al., 1987). We aren't (and never have been) a single thing but are probably better thought of as a collection of inter-related, living processes, experiences and responses (a multiplicity) ceaselessly interacting with aspects of ourselves and the world around us in a constant becoming. Successful identities, then, are probably not a finish line that is crossed when we, with a Marie Kondo-like capacity, finally have everything about us in its right place, but rather when we are able to maintain some sort of stable balance within the constant changes of identity (Bateson, 1972a). Somewhat akin to a lumberjack staying upright by constantly adjusting to the movement of the floating log he's standing on, a stable identity results from the connection between many processes and reflective responses enabling the right adjustments at the right time.

A second key aspect of identity is that it is something that is ours, and (in many cultures) that the independent quality of our experience is a key virtue of what our identity includes. Systems thinking, however, would suggest that our connection to others is changeable and incompletely recognised but ultimately unavoidable. We might value the notion of our independence and our freedom, but we also value the real and practical way that we belong with and to others, even if we find this challenging (Castells, 1997). We feel we belong within our families, communities, societies, tribes and groups, some, ironically enough, feeling kinship and solidarity through their focused reassertion of their independence and their freedom. We explore and express how we belong with other people in all sorts of ways, even through our appreciation of our participation in systems as consumers (Bauman & May, 2001; Keat et al., 1994). While we can rely on our connections with others being a feature of our experience, the connections themselves change frequently. Relationships grow and wither. Some do so as a feature of their temporary nature. My systemic connection with a person whom I meet providing tech support over a phone line is brief by design but our interaction still constitutes a small, temporary social system. Beliefs and values including those about social ideals (systems of meaning) such as family or nationhood; how we prioritise maintaining connections; and the value we place on specific relationships are not static, and relationships may change accordingly (Bauman, 2004b). Newer modes of communication and connection such as social media are responses to changes and instruments of change. There was reason to hope that social media might achieve our wish to be more immediately connected to others, and every reason to believe that its use hasn't made us feel closer or feel more confident in our identities (Hargreaves, 2003).[40] Other types of social systems such as economic and legal systems also have similar characteristics. We may not feel we are constantly communicating with these systems but if we do need to communicate economically (buying something) or legally (signing a contract) engaging with systems which include this communication, as changeable and multi-faceted as they are, is unavoidable.

A natural response to any acceptance that systems (and our identity) are contributed to by many processes and are constantly shifting and changing would be to wonder: what causes this to happen? Systems change due to "perturbations". Perturbations are simply the forces and processes, internal or external which create change within systems (Wang, 2013). While perturbations are experienced within a system, they are often themselves the result of changes within other inter-connected systems. That is, there is a process of inter-system reconciliation, from which each system determines its own results. My eyes appreciate changing light triggering transmission of messages. These are interpreted by the visual centre of my brain as a set of images: it is getting dark and raining outside. Other memory and motivational cognitive systems associate these perceptions with the awareness that I have to pick up my son. This influences nerve and motor systems to hoist me out of my chair and away from the keyboard toward the car. Each step within this chain involves interpretation and influence of another system which perturbs them into responding. However, different images may not have done so. If my visual system had appreciated that it was bright and sunny, the chain of influences would have stopped quickly, Or, if my memory and motivational systems had responded to the perturbing images of rain and darkness with the reassuring memory that my wife was already on the way to school, the images would have ceased to induce change in the systems and the cascade of influences would have ceased. Similarly, if my wife had been standing beside me saying, "it's time you picked up our son" the result of my sprinting to the car may have been the same, but the involvement of the visual systems in bringing this about would have been minimal as sound is not a communication that they can receive. Living systems, by their structure, elements and communication, determine what perturbs them and how they will respond.

Thinking further about what might perturb or influence the systems contributing to identity, we might start to get a sense of how complex this can be. What is understood as a person's identity is a multitude of different perspectives, beliefs, experiences and values interacting as an amalgam. This means that how an identity is appreciated from within different mental and social systems may reflect rich, yet diverse meanings, many of which may not be easily appreciated by us. For example, self-identifying as an Indigenous Australian is an experience that I, as a white Australian male, have arguably no authority to be able to describe or, potentially, understand. However, this statement, and my feeling that including it is necessary already begins to indicate how complex the systems and influences which are involved in Indigenous Australian identities might be. Australian Indigenous culture has been described as including a worldview that balances the outer space of "country" and the inner space of experience within a cyclical understanding of the passage of time (Brady, 1994: 14). This is an ancient and unique system of experience arising and developing from the coupling of many systems of thinking, belief, story, meaning, community, and living with and within the land over millennia. Changes in these stable connections have occurred, but slowly, meaning that Indigenous culture, as understood by those who do, has been relatively robust. The relationship of this view to contemporary Indigenous Australian culture and identity is nonetheless contested and understood in diverse ways. More recent influences on Indigenous culture and identity, including colonisation, conflict, massacres and systemic violence, the stolen generations, land rights, stigma and systemic racism, mainstream educational and health responses to Indigenous people, and responses to attempts at self-determination, the *Uluru Statement from the Heart* and the unsuccessful Voice referendum of 2023 are elements of the dramatic perturbations of what contributes to and what it means to identify as Indigenous in Australia (Andersen, 2019; Grieves, 2014; Morris, 2018). These and many other influences on Indigenous identity and culture, sustained, continuing and episodic

— from more recently coupled systems compared with those central in the previous millennia — have had a dynamic impact resulting in more apparent and immediate change. What it means to identify as an Indigenous person would always have been something that was developing and influenced by multiple systems, but those changes have been more dramatic, tragic and observable from outside that culture since colonisation.

While the question of Australian Aboriginal identity is a highly complex example, it serves to demonstrate that what we understand as our identity often arises from tensions between systems. Bauman suggests that the experience of identity emerges from the tension between those identities that may be assigned to us by others and ourselves (Bauman, 2004b). Our experience of our identity is the results of reconciling how we see ourselves with how we are seen by others. If identity is a process of reconciliation of systems of meaning and experience, then the dualities of dependence and independence, or belonging and being an outcast, are all valid elements of how we fit (have structurally coupled) ourselves to our world. Although some may shun the frail, the mad, and the dying, it is ultimately the human frailties of our body, mind and circumstance that bind us all together (Lingis 1994). These frailties are awkward and uncomfortable contributors to all identities whether we accept them or not. The nothingness that death represents and that we all have in common, is, for Lingis, the portal through which we can access an understanding that we truly belong with others (Lingis, 1994). We interpret our world, present ourselves to our world and are also connected to our world through the physical systems of our body and the social systems of our communication (Merleau-Ponty & Smith, 2005). As frail and changing systems, we live and grow and dissolve over time. As Agich reminds us, "the body stand(s) in complex dialogue with the world primarily through movement and activity", and it is through that dialogue that we affect the systems while those systems that we experience as "us" are also being affected (Agich, 1993a). For all of us, including persons with dementia, our identities and our appreciation of others arise in response to the interconnection of the personal systems of human experience and the environments that surround them, including the presence of others and the broader influences of our culture and language.

Systems and decisions

It makes sense that the things that I decide are related at least some of the time to who I think I am. When we decide to buy this rather than that, we do it for some reason. The reason may not be particularly deep or resonant, for instance, the product I buy (say a box of Frosted Krusty O's cereal) may be slightly closer on the shelf, or it may have a slightly more attractive box. But some choices might be for reasons that adhere to something important to us, such as that the product is better for the environment or that its affordability is attractive due to our need to budget. Systems thinking provides us with tools to help explain how these elements of decision-making fit together. Thinking and talking about decisions can be seen as an assertion and reinforcement of who we think we are but also as a process of experimenting and trying out ideas and testing them against our perception of ourselves. A field of systems thinking called cybernetics tells us that, while I feel that I am indeed choosing the Krusty O's, what is actually happening is that I'm also being steered away from all the other choices that are being ruled out, in a process technically called restraint (Bateson, 1972a). A choice does not occur because there is only one right option but because multiple options that don't fit the situation are ruled out, like the incorrect pieces of a jigsaw puzzle that our hand passes over. Processes of restraint can also be perceived in our self-expression through the choices we make in language. In choosing to use the word "sharp" to describe the feeling of the Krusty O's in my mouth I am ruling out inappropriate words such as "soft", or "crunchy". However, using the word "sharp" to describe what I'm feeling also exposes restraint from other systems. My mental and perceptual systems and the external features of the object itself work together to restrain the possible choices to express my understanding of this experience towards the singular idea of "sharp". It is not just a matter of a choice of the right word, but reconciliation across systems that restrain me towards an option. Often the result of this reconciliation will be a decision that is "not wrong" as much as it is "right" and developing restraints is a process of trial and error (Bateson, 1972a). I learn which visual perceptions and linguistic symbols don't mean "tree" or "dog" or "jagged metal" as I become more confident in my ability to determine whether I'm perceiving these things. Such a refining of options, a mental process that is below awareness, underlies all choices so that what seems realistically available and apparent to a person is pruned by this process. This contributes to more predictable and stable systemic processes, where the most likely choices are the ones that have been chosen before. Ultimately, this demonstrates how the inter-system processes of winnowing out "wrong" options (restraint) leads to more predictable and frequent choices (sometimes called habituation) and are seeds of what we perceive of as identity. Identity, a developed and shared sense of who we are, becomes clearer to us and to others through a continuity of choices and approaches to problems for a person (or a community) that are meaningful and self-reinforcing to them.

Such a view of decision-making and its implications for identity, as a process based on the inter-connection of systems, is also valid for social systems. While the framing of the decisions (described above) has related to individuals, systemic processes also restrain and habituate choices within groups of people and through communication. People's communication works within often somewhat invisible cooperative agreements where we feel we mean certain things when we communicate certain things. When I say that a Krusty O feels jagged and metallic in my mouth when I try to eat it, you might be surprised but you also have a sense of what that means. It is the success of understanding which is critical (Habermas 1990). Speech is understood and communication achieved when those involved feel that they understand what was meant and why it was said even if these elements aren't stated. This often requires discussion and exploration to test the reasons underlying positions, seeking to ascertain whether they are sincere, right and true (Bohman & Rehg, 2007). Understanding others and making decisions to agree and cooperate with them are thus determined by complex systems of social and communicative factors. Jurgen Habermas has described how all of this takes place in practice with his concept of the "lifeworld".

Habermas's concept of the lifeworld was an important component of his theory of "communicative action" (Habermas, 1990). The lifeworld referred both to communications resulting in shared understanding and the context and resources that enable this communicative connection. From his perspective, the lifeworld is a shared space of meaning and cultural significance. Because we participate in the vastness of the lifeworld, like the horizon, our view of it is partial and influenced by where we're standing. The lifeworld is also not static but is constantly shifting due to the participation of us all (Finlayson, 2005). The way we connect, communicate, argue and understand through our shared lifeworld constantly disturbs or perturbs it while also acting as a kind of "repair-work" where we fashion it into new things (Habermas, 1990). It is through our communication and our interpretation within the context of systems like our culture and our language that we shape our shared view of our world with others.

We can say that the interactions between personal, social and cultural systems are expressed through decision-making, represent and give rise to our identities, and occur due to our relationships with others. Decisions are shared acts of communication that ripple out with influence, affecting many other systems. Such acts of communication construct and explore meanings and connections between individuals through the interpretation of their world around them. This "process of definition and re-definition", of contribution to the shared lifeworld, contains the shared contexts that underlie the cohesion (and the turbulence) of our relationships and our communities (Habermas, 1990). Identity similarly arises as a representation of the person, which is explored and delineated through communication in the context of multiple interdependent personal and social systems. Decision-making, identity, relationships and the lived experience of networks of people are all fundamental expressions of the interaction of human systems. These ideas seem to cast the "problems" of dementia in an entirely new light, which we'll explore further in the next chapter.

2. Systems in dementia

As we explored at the beginning of Part Three, systems thinking brings new ways of approaching the multiple challenges in dementia. Systems thinking ideas aren't completely new to thinking through what dementia means and how to best provide care to people who've been affected by it. Research to try to learn lessons from systems thinking and adapt our understanding and approach to dementia has been underway for some time. Much of this work does not refer explicitly to systems thinking as I've discussed it but does resonate strongly with it.

Social systems, for instance, have been an increasing and influential area of focus in dementia care and research for several decades. Such research has often brought in the views or presence of a "third person", often a spouse or family member who was deeply involved in the healthcare of the person with dementia, in response to an awareness that such voices are important and historically silent. This "triadic" view has evolved from the work of Simmel who described patterns of behaviour within triads (of a "patient", a clinician and an important other person) that affect how these relationships work (Simmel, 1950). Developing these ideas led to some complex interactions being recognised as contributors to "pathology" and potentially as targets for therapy within approaches like family therapy and "relationship-centred care" in dementia (Adams & Gardiner, 2005). Triadic networks remain a common and influential idea to support research and care in dementia. Models such as the "triadic interaction", "partnership approach" and the "Senses Framework" in dementia care are based on this way of understanding the importance of networks of people in the experience of dementia (Fortinsky, 2001; Nolan, Brown, et al., 2006; Nolan et al., 2002).

Triadic approaches to exploring and supporting dementia care have focused particularly on exploring the dynamics of support provided to persons with dementia, especially from family members (B. A. Elliott et al., 2007; Lieberman & Fisher, 1999). These approaches define the dementia experience as relating to and resulting from how these triadic relationships work. However, they do not usually define these relationships as social systems or dig further into the other interacting systems that might be important contributors to how triads work. For example, Adams' influential "relationship-centred care" identifies communication within networks of people as a key determinant of the dementia experience and is highly influenced by family systems therapy as an approach to improve this kind of care for people with dementia (Adams & Gardiner, 2005). Adams sees the social presence of the person with dementia as being enabled or disabled by how others around the person with dementia communicate and position themselves bodily. It follows that a skilled approach to how we talk and how we are around people with dementia will limit the systemic contributors to diminishing the person with dementia's social and communicative presence. However, this approach adopts a fairly narrow systemic view of dementia, as it focuses on these close relationships without including the broader systemic contribution (through language and culture for instance) to how these smaller systems operate. Nolan's use of the Senses Framework for relationship-centred care provides another example (Nolan, Brown, et al., 2006). This model's focus on six "senses": "security", "belonging", "continuity", "purpose", "achievement" and "significance" which, it suggests, should be optimised to achieve the best care, provides clear therapeutic direction for aged care staff and a greater recognition of the contribution of residents and families to care outcomes than is possible from a person-centred approach to care (Nolan, Davies, et al., 2006). This framework is a valuable contribution which supports the creation of environments and interactions that allow "everyone to grow". Nolan's Senses and, in particular, further work on these ideas from Watson also highlight the extension of the networks beyond individual clinicians to groups within institutions and the institutions themselves, that is, the idea that broader social systems than just those "around the bedside" need to be considered in this kind of work (Watson, 2019). But in all these cases, the attention to the implications of systems thinking in dementia is largely focused on social interaction, and primarily on clinical care support. These approaches largely accept that the diagnosis of dementia and the experience of the person with dementia themselves exist as independent "things" rather than, as we've explored, experiences and ideas which are arising from the interaction of multiple different systems.

• • •

Further research helps us refine a systems thinking approach to understanding dementia by exploring the interaction between social and mental systems for persons with dementia. An important example is the work of Steven Sabat. Sabat describes how the inter-relationship of mental and social systems leads to several different inter-related selves for people with dementia (Sabat, 2002). In his model, Self 1 is the self of a singular and consistent personal identity (how we know ourselves); Self 2 is the self of mental and physical attributes, past and present (our appearance, what we believe, and what we have thought and done); and Self 3 is the multiplicity of social identities that the person constructs with the necessary cooperation of others (our social and public identity). In identifying these elements, Sabat suggests that our social selves (Self 3) are at greatest risk from dementia. However, changes in our social selves can also affect how people with dementia (and others) interpret and focus on the characteristics of a person with dementia (Self 2) with more attention to aspects which support the common "burdensome, dysfunctional patient" idea of people with dementia.

Sabat's work provides useful descriptions of elements or domains of identity for people with dementia and how changes in one area can affect another. Sabat's approach also shows us how difficult it is as an observer to define identity. One challenge is the natural intuitive attention we tend to place on what a person *has* been when we're considering identity. Bauman refers to this as a kind of "nostalgia" on the part of an observer (Bauman, 2004b). Sabat's descriptions of the elements of self identify the person with dementia relative to their past, who they have been, and roles that they had: the selves of people with dementia are considered nostalgically so that their belonging and their identity arise through a static link to their past. But it is important to note here that Sabat didn't just decide this was a good idea. His position is based on empirical work with people with dementia, for example, the explanation from a person with dementia that they "(are) still a lawyer" (Sabat & Harré, 1992). Sabat feels that we are on firmer ground in determining that there is more value in a person with dementia's links to their historical self than in affirming or supporting the more current identities of people with dementia (Sabat, 2002). This is an understandable and common view. Comments from dementia networks in Part Two of this book also often shared a similar focus. If not more valid, it is at least easier to try to understand people with dementia by focusing on who they've been rather than on who they are now. In Part One, I discussed Tom Kitwood's work that drew attention to how what we think about dementia and how we talk and act around people with dementia plays a big role in creating their experience and expectations. In different ways, both Sabat and Kitwood remind us that *remembering who a person with dementia was* is important. The historical identity and their status as a person are important contributors to who the person with dementia is now. Said in another way, having a diagnosis of dementia doesn't remove our connection to all that we once were. However, holding on to unchanged aspects of our beliefs and our physicality as self-defining also seems to create an expectation that our selves and identities shouldn't change. It suggests that without dementia, the person's self would have remained an unchanged and valued continuity. You can see where this is heading: namely, that any change to the robustness of this historical identity is automatically a loss to the current person. This perspective sets us up to interpret common changes of dementia in a predetermined way as a tragic dismantling of an identity. However, as we saw from the conversations with dementia networks, while this was a common perspective it wasn't the only one. Dementia networks acknowledged how change in identity could also include growth, acceptance and transcendence, for instance. However, focusing on who we've been as the most important value makes it difficult to view the changes to identity in dementia as anything other than loss. Using systems thinking to engage with this challenge suggests another perspective and opens up more possible interpretations. Systems thinking would suggest that identity is a reflective, ceaseless process contributed to by many systems. Systems thinking seems to create space for a person with dementia to retain a valid identity even if it is vastly different from how things used to be.

A systems view of a dementia network

To begin to start to think through the implications of systems thinking for dementia further, we need a place to start. Probably the easiest place to do this is to start with the dementia networks themselves, since (as we discussed above) there's already been some movement toward recognising the importance of this relational, systems thinking approach to engaging with the challenges of dementia. It's also arguably a little easier to think about how systems thinking might apply to how we are together than it is to think about how it applies to how an individual thinks and feels. So, let's start by using systems thinking to describe the social system of the dementia network and see where that takes us.

To summarise a few points from our previous discussions, to begin with we'd be accepting that the world is essentially constructed, or arising from systems, not in isolation but interconnected to each other in complex ways through their boundaries. A "social system" is a particular kind of system which is made up of communicative processes whose function is to ensure their own continuity (i.e. to continue working as a system). There are different types of social systems but they share qualities of being able to change and respond to changes in function and interaction with their environment — which would include human systems like the mental and physical systems of a person. Any system can be described based on what it's made of, how those parts interact, and how it's able to change. Based on these ideas we're now in a position to think through how these ideas might apply to the networks of people with dementia.

The following sections are going to try and dig into both how you can "see" a dementia network as a living, social system and how you can use that information to try to learn more about how that network is working and what sorts of things seem to be a challenge for it. It is going to get a little bit technical. If you want to cut to the chase and find out more about what I learned, rather than how I learned it, feel free to skip to the chapter "Mapping change in dementia systems".

The structure and function of a dementia network

Maturana describes several elements that must be present for something to be a living system. An important element is that living systems have changeable structures while still retaining organisation (H. R. Maturana, 1974). A cycling team may, over time, change its riders, its coach and its manager but it will still be involved in the primary function of being a cycling team and considered the "same" team despite the changes. More pointedly, all the cells in a person's body may change over time and yet they remain part of the same person. The different cells still work in largely the same way, enough at least for us to say that the person is still alive in the same way. The person still has an unchanged purpose (fundamentally, to continue to be alive and function as a system), it still needs its connection with its environment for sustenance and interaction, it still is the "same" system despite changes to what it's made of (components) and how they interact together (connections). This unchanged purpose is not necessarily a single thing — a cycling team may have a purpose of continuing to be a cycling team, to win multiple grand tours, and attract attention to their sponsors among other things — but this purpose or function remains a coherent aspect of the living system.

What does this all mean for dementia networks? Let's break it down and discuss the various structures of a dementia network.

Function and components

As we have described, social systems are defined by a network of components, or nodes, with links of communication between them. For the network with persons with dementia, the nodal points of these networks are communicative aspects of those people who are involved. These might be best thought of as events as they are not fixed but occur and contribute to a system at a particular moment. Luhmann did write about systems relating to healthcare but his work focused on how big, pervasive social systems (for instance the health architecture of a country) respond to a person being well or sick (Gibson & Boiko, 2012). While this has some relevance to how our society might see people with dementia in the broad sense, it's a little less helpful when thinking about the smaller, likely dynamic structures around a person with dementia. Based on what we heard from our dementia networks, they often seem to have a focus on care. This doesn't seem surprising given the context of their situation. We're on relatively safe ground in proposing the function of these dementia networks as being about the care and support of people with dementia. By doing this we're narrowing in on what we're primarily interested in. While everyone with a connection to the person with dementia is in some way contributing to their social systems, the important component events (and people doing them) that interest us are those involved in care. We could therefore say that what this network is, is a care system of people with dementia.

Being involved in this care system doesn't imply a role or title, but rather making a real contribution. A family doctor who has been involved in providing medical support to a family for 30 years, but who becomes less involved might not significantly contribute to the ongoing care events for the social system of a person with dementia, while a newly met neighbour may contribute something very meaningful by bringing in the bins, the mail and the laundry. From our work with people with dementia, this usually involves the person with the diagnosis themselves, friends or family members who are "carers" and paid care staff who might include doctors, nurses, aged care workers and others. In commenting that persons contribute to the components of the system, we also recognise that a "person" is not equivalent to a component in a social system. Only the person's contribution to a care event are aspects of this system. Each person in the network has numerous systems which all interact to making up that person, including their physical systems and their mental processes. All of these interact with and are required for communication, but it is only the communicative aspects of that person that participates within the care system of the person with dementia. No one system can contain a whole "person" or "self" given all the bits that make it up, and so that person or self in totality can't contribute to a single system. It's also important to add that when we say communication here, we're not limited to speech or writing. Valid communication within a care network of a person with dementia would include acts of physical or social care like helping a person to shower or taking them shopping. Noting this also highlights that the components of a social care system in dementia and the people involved in contributing those components will change (with changing care needs for a person with dementia over time). This has two components in that new people might become involved in a network due to a need for new care communication, for instance a family member becoming involved in taking a parent for a coffee as an outing every week, or that communication components may be maintained with different people involved, say if the family member wasn't available and so a volunteer took a person with dementia for an outing.

Connections

The connections between these events, the things that turn these potentially random moments into something that we can describe as a system, boil down to the notion of communication. Luhmann argues that communication involves three cardinal elements: information, utterance and understanding, and all three are needed to be present for communication to occur (Luhmann, 1992). Using the example of economics, in a restaurant I announce that I'm ready to pay my bill by pushing back from the table and placing my cutlery on my plate. My smile and nod inform the staff that I am indeed ready to pay, and there's a mutual understanding that now comes the moment for payment when the staff will announce to me how much I owe them. Within the language of care, a person with dementia might announce that they feel things are getting harder for them. They inform others that they want more help, and those in the care network understand from the message that more must be done, or that explanations of the limits of what can be done are required. All of these aspects are dependent on the context and what's meaningful to the care system. What's meant by "understanding" is particularly important and challenging in the context of a problem like dementia where communication changes are common. It's often assumed that people with more advanced dementia can't communicate or are unable to understand what is being conveyed to them. When we observe that communication in dementia has changed to the point of being unrecognisable in comparison to what preceded, does that mean communication is impossible? I don't think so. Even when we're not easily able to interpret a person with dementia's responses to their experiences, it seems possible, at least for some people some of the time, that communication can take place. Perhaps we need to adopt the right lens or approach to interpretation, but understanding *can* be possible. Persons with dementia are actively and responsively engaged with their experiences even if the interpretation of their responses requires more patience, curiosity, creativity and being comfortable with ambiguity than is usually afforded (Chapman et al., 2022).

System dynamics — perturbations and change

Thinking through the components and connections of a dementia system provides some sense of the structure, which is important. It's hard to understand a system without understanding what it's made of. But systems are constantly changing, and thinking of systems as static structures also won't really help us to understand what's going on. To do that we really need to dig further into how system change happens. Before we start thinking through how this applies to dementia networks let's walk through some of the key ideas in general terms. Systems by definition respond to change and their environment. A way of conceptualising this is through identifying the things that tend to influence and lead to change in a system, let's call these perturbations (H. R. Maturana, 1974). There are a few different ways of thinking about what can perturb a system. One way is that perturbations can be triggered from within the system by some kind of internal process. The developing skills of a cyclist in our cycling team leading to the team changing roster might be an example of this. They can also be triggered by changes from outside. A change in the rules governing cycling teams and how many riders they're allowed to have that leads to a similar change in roster might be an example of this. However, in both these cases and regardless of where the trigger for the changes starts the changes in response to the perturbation are the system's perturbations (i.e. they come from the system) as the system is involved in internally communicating or making sense of these influences once they've arrived. Returning to our discussion of the person buying a coffee, this economic system might, for instance, be affected by something outside it, say a natural disaster in Costa Rica leading to less coffee being available. This outside change wouldn't have a direct impact on the small economic system of a person buying a coffee but might indirectly lead to changes that the system can make sense of — likely as a higher price for the coffee. Systems determine how they respond to influences. For social systems though, responses are through the mechanism of communication (Luhmann, 2014a). This also means that how social systems respond to perturbations through communication indicates to us what can influence the system and what changes have resulted (Dell, 1985). If I finish drinking my coffee at iCafe and I signal that I'm ready to pay for my coffee and the waiter understands me and tells me that it will cost $6, the price and expectation from that waiter won't change because I say that it used to be $4 or if I try to leave without paying. Those aren't likely to be effective ways to communicate and induce change within that system. So, systems can be triggered to respond by things from inside or outside them, but noticing what they seem to respond to and how they respond to it can allow us to describe how change occurs in that system and what the system responds (or is sensitive) to.

Now let's turn our attention to thinking through these ideas in relation to dementia systems. It makes intuitive, and perhaps self-evident, sense that a significant influence on the social systems of persons with dementia is dementia itself. Dementia has a complex impact on dementia networks as social systems. For instance, it impacts a multitude of environmental systems that are external to and support the social system. We'll discuss this in more detail later, but an obvious example is that dementia has an impact on the cognitive or mental systems of the person with dementia which leads to lots of other social impacts. Dementia also affects the components of the social system of a dementia network. It results in new people becoming part of the system for new reasons, such as new healthcare providers and care providers becoming involved in providing care to the person with dementia. It also affects communication within the social system, for instance, because of the challenges in recognising, interpreting and understanding attempts at communication due to dementia. Dementia is, in this sense, a complex of challenges to the social system, an influence which perturbs this social system from within and without.

Importantly, the nature of the system as a responsive entity means that a degree of change (easily observable or otherwise) is unavoidable. The social system of the dementia network just has to change because of the dementia. Systems are changing all the time anyway, and so the question really is not, is change happening, but what kind, and why? Therefore, uncovering the perturbations that we know are happening gives us a chance to understand and map the kinds of changes that are constantly occurring and figure out what sort of impact they are all having. While we can be confident that perturbations will occur and will affect the system, how they do this and what changes result will be specific and contextual. It's also timely to remind ourselves that the result of all of these changes, on one level, is how dementia is experienced for those people who make up the dementia network. Again, however, it is dementia itself which is very likely a major influence on the changes happening within the systems of the network. And so, dementia is what is experienced by the people within the network, but dementia also changes or "transforms" not only what that experience is but what that experience is built up from and consists of (Komesaroff, 2008b). It might be worth reflecting on that again for a second, because it feels like an important point. Dementia is not a single or a series of predictable problems. Rather, it seems to set in place a cascade of changes within the systems which we are all made up of and, ultimately, has impacts upon the deeply significant parts of experience like our sense of identity, our relationships and the experience of being ourselves.

Using systems in dementia

Hopefully, at this point, we're all convinced that systems thinking seems a useful idea for starting to think through some of the complex problems that we've identified in dementia. But we still need to establish whether there's something useful that comes out of that information. Ultimately, the hope is for something within all of these ideas that can make dementia easier or less difficult for those on whom the diagnosis has an impact. We still seem to be some way from that at this point, so let's think through what comes next.

In the research with dementia networks that gave rise to this book, I used the systems thinking ideas we've started to discuss to try to understand in a new way the stories that I'd heard from people with dementia, their carers and their healthcare providers. The next chapter will discuss what I found from doing that, but at this point I want to say a little bit more about how I did that and why. As we discussed above, the key idea here is that, if dementia networks are social systems, then the communication those networks shared, the stories, feelings, descriptions and explanations they told me would include information about what sorts of changes were happening within these systems and what was triggering those changes. Trying to figure that out was a process of working through and hearing what sorts of factors and forces seemed important to explain those stories when thinking about the network as an interconnected community rather than a group of individual people.

Doing this required many different steps which built one upon the other. I tried to break down what I heard and learned from people in dementia networks into small parts, and I tried to build those parts into a whole and tried to see what the parts could tell us about the whole and vice versa (Gharajedaghi & Ackoff, 1984). I read and thought about what resulted from all of this poring over the words of these networks to see what seemed most important. I identified what I thought people in the network were trying to communicate to each other and then tried to check whether this seemed to be what was being understood by others (Gibson & Boiko, 2012). I also looked at all of what I'd heard from people with dementia and their networks and tried to see if I could find links between what seemed generally important to them as a big group of people (say, the big group of all the people with dementia or all the carers that I talked to), and what seemed important to those small networks of people. Finally, I also tried to map out what seemed to be perturbing and influencing these networks (based on all of the work above) and then used these ideas to examine what sorts of changes seemed to be taking place within dementia networks as a result.

In trying to map perturbations within a system it is important to remember that there are relationships between what perturbs and influences a system and the communication that results. The coffee price doesn't go up by chance because of a disaster in Costa Rica, there is a relationship between this initial event and each subsequent link in the chain of events. Similarly, if you can get to the heart of what people in dementia networks express about what they felt was challenging, impactful and meaningful about their experiences this seemed very likely to relate to the sorts of things that had influenced and perturbed their care system. I say very likely here because, of course, living systems are incredibly complex and it is difficult to be confident about the details of why everything works out in one particular way. However, working backwards like this from already knowing what those in the network were saying about what was important and trying to use this to figure out how that related to what was influencing the systems and making change, we could be a little more confident that we were on the right track.

Systems change all the time, but they tend to change in some characteristic kinds of ways. Knowing this when I was working through what the systems seemed to be influenced by allowed me to describe what sorts of change seemed to be happening in the networks. Let's work through this with some questions. If systems are changing all the time, then what kind of things are changing? Well, as we mentioned the structure and the connections can all be changing but really what this all comes down to is stability. What happens to the stability of the system as a result of a perturbation is really the core outcome when you're thinking this through (Bateson, 1972a; Meadows, 2008). We're going to focus on two kinds of changes in the dementia networks corresponding to different effects on the stability of the system that have resulted from the perturbations. One change type happens when a perturbation results in fairly limited changes in the components, communication or function of the care network, such as that it seems that the change is a balancing or stabilising force to return to a largely stable or business as usual point. We can call this first-order change (Fraser, 2007). If, however, the perturbation and response lead to more radical instability and transformative change in the system then this is usually described as a second-order change (Barker & Chang, 2013; Parmenidou, 2011).

At this point, you might also be wondering whether this means that there's a good type of change and a bad one. I mean, it sounds like a change from a perturbation which doesn't rock the boat much is a good one, and one which leads to more radical transformation is bad, right? Well, unfortunately it's not quite that simple. Different situations can make either of these change types good or bad for a system in the sense of making the system function better or worse. It depends on what's going on. We'll discuss this in more detail later after we've worked through some examples, but it's probably fair at this point just to note that it depends on the context of that particular system at that time whether either of these changes will be good or bad for the system.

Bringing all of these ideas together, both for the analysis that I've described above and for this book, required creating stories. Using and generating stories to make sense of complicated human experiences follows a long and important tradition (Charon, 2006). The logic here is that when we hear, interpret and re-tell stories (particularly when we are being open and honest about doing so) we are not saying that this is the only "true" way of understanding that story, but we are letting that story "breathe" (using the words of Arthur Frank) and demonstrating that a story has some validity and power because it has an impact on us as readers and on us as story-tellers (Frank, 2010a). I used what people with dementia, their carers and their health carers shared with me and brought it all together into stories. These stories, developed from talking to dementia networks, were a way of exploring what they had to tell and helping to convey those messages in a meaningful way (Ely et al., 1997; Spalding & Phillips, 2007). You've already encountered parts of these stories earlier in the book. I've used them as a way of tying the ideas that we've explored back into the everyday human experience of people on whose lives dementia has a significant impact. In the chapter below we're going to explore some more of these stories, but we'll focus specifically on these questions of what seems to perturb dementia networks and what sorts of changes can be detected as a result.

3. Mapping change in dementia systems

Trying to map what's occurring in any living system is a very complex task. It ends up being a balance of stating the mundane and obvious and claiming insight into things that are very difficult to be confident about. It's difficult to feel completely confident of what's happening within groups of people like dementia networks. Like all living systems, the networks are constantly changing. Any judgement or conclusion we come to by careful thinking is, by definition, already out of date because it's based on information from how things used to be, not how they are now. This is particularly true of this chapter where the stories that we will think through together have already happened. They are in the past. In effect, these stories are about systems and people that have already moved on. However, we can still gain much insight from these stories that might be relevant to other networks right now. With beings as interesting as people, particularly around the time of the huge life changes that dementia usually involves, it is also unlikely that there is only a single relevant perturbation in any affected system. Even considering the relatively simple system of the nerve and muscle control required for me to hit these keys when I intend to requires an intricate balance of impulses, mechanics, pressures and counter-pressures to keep the whole process on track — not a single, solitary perturbation. Given all of this, it's important for me to say again that, in this chapter, I'm not claiming to have some kind of special insight that others don't have, that I *really* know what's going on for dementia networks. Instead, this chapter is about exploring the ideas that seem important to dementia networks, what we can detect when we're tuning in to what the dementia network is telling us is influencing it and what seems to be happening in response. It also seems fair to say and assume that within dementia networks, dementia itself will be a major force for change and that anything else that seems to be influencing the network will be doing so within a backdrop of dementia's influence. Let's be clear that what is to be discussed in this section is not a comprehensive account of all that could be said, but a workable start to thinking through the sorts of influences which might be important in dementia networks when change is occurring.

You may be wondering why this would be useful to know. Perhaps we're willing to accept that common types of perturbation can be detected, but in what way would this helpful? We'll spend more time working through this but, in essence, the answer here is that, if we know more about what triggers networks to change, we'll know more about what's led to them being in the (often difficult) pattern of responses that they're currently in. Also, if the sorts of influences that we can detect can perturb and trigger change in dementia networks, there seems to be the tantalising possibility that similar sorts of factors might be able to be used to influence dementia networks positively and therapeutically.

From my research with dementia networks there are five major types of perturbing factors or challenges which seem to influence how networks change and adapt. These seem to fit, in turn, into three categories. I'll discuss each of the factors as part of one of these categories — which are: "how we are together", which is all about how those in the dementia network connect with each other; "how we are individually", which is all about what separates and defines individual members of the network; and "our perception", which is all about what dementia is like for the dementia networks. The first two factors which seem to have a big influence on what's happening within the dementia networks come from the first group, "how we are together". These factors are *relationships*, and *status and power*. In the second group "how we are individually", there seemed to be one major influential factor which was *identity*. The final group mentioned above, "our perception", included how dementia influenced *current experiences* and the *future*.

Each of these perturbing factors seemed to relate to and help explain how dementia networks responded to what was happening for them. As we've noted, it's fair to say that these factors likely weren't the only thing that was influencing the systems, but they were observable factors which made sense in explaining what seemed to be occurring. In what follows I'll be sharing stories which hopefully make this clear, but in each case these factors seemed helpful in explaining change in multiple different networks. In these stories these perturbing factors seemed to lead to different types of change. These changes are best understood as the responses of the system to these influences: what the system did when these influences made their impact. Two types of change were evident: stabilising (first-order) or transforming (second order) responses. Which of these occurred depended on the system itself.

In the following sections we'll explore some stories to learn more about what they can tell us about the factors which influenced networks and how this led to change. In the writing and analysis of these sections the text will often simplify some of the ideas we've explored in systems thinking. For instance, it will talk about "Fred's" responses or what "Fred felt ..." when we are really meaning that "Fred's communication indicated ...". As we've discussed it is not the whole person but the communication they contribute to a social system that marks their involvement in that system. However, for ease of reading, the text will associate what has been done or said with a whole person.

How we are together

How the people within the dementia network connected to each other and their sense of their bonds and links to others often seemed to be a key factor influencing the social system. In the examples below this was associated with relationships, what they mean to people and how they change, and notions of status and power within care systems and how that influenced system functions. Relationships seemed a challenge for dementia networks due to new demands and pressures, particularly when this was in the context of relationships where there was already a degree of fraying or deterioration. Experiences like significant loss, bereavement, distrust and anger could all have an impact upon and add to the impact of these challenges. Status and power challenges often seemed related to the influence of changing authority and roles within care systems. Things like people being involved in care roles which felt unwanted or unnatural were examples of these kinds of contributing factors.

Relationships

The sense of relationships, what they meant and what sorts of changes were felt to have happened or might happen in the future could all be experienced by those within the dementia networks. These sorts of experiences influenced how the network members continued in relationships with each other — with effects for the change and stability of those network communities. Let's start exploring the impact of relationships on dementia care networks with a story from Mary's care network.

Mary's care network's story

I met Mary in a hospice palliative care unit. She looked tiny, sitting forward in an oversize hospital lounge chair, often speaking so softly that I needed to concentrate hard to catch each word. She'd been in the hospice for about a week at that point and for about a month in hospital prior to that. The move to the hospice was in response to her health slowly getting worse and the absence of a clear plan for her to be able to be anywhere else. Mary seemed weak and frail, but also comfortable where she was. She'd had dementia for many years. It was familiar to her and she seemed comfortable with it. Mary's dementia had affected her recollection of her stories and also her place in them, but that wasn't a bother to her. "I am just me," she would say with an enigmatic glint in her eye when you tried to uncover what all that meant to her. The only thing I ever felt confident about was that Mary's real focus wasn't herself, it was others.

Mary's relationships were the key to how she felt about everything, about moving to the hospice, about her future and her past. For Mary, this wasn't a change. She couldn't recall a time when it had ever been different. Her connection to her family, her God, were a deep source of meaning. It wasn't just that these relationships were important or strong but, from Mary's perspective, they expressed something fundamental about how people get along. Every relationship she could recall with people from her past had this precious sense for her. They revealed something ideal: the fabric of which relationships are made. Even newer relationships, like those with the staff around her, resonated with meaning for Mary and they, from her perspective, had always done so. She felt understood and loved by the "kind" people who care for her, and so loved them in return. Surrounded by such "lovely" people, Mary felt confident that she must have wanted to come to the palliative care unit; how could it be otherwise? She loved the staff there so much that now the unit was her "second home".

Feeling this kindness from others made Mary want to be kinder, too. She also hoped that being kinder would support others around her to reciprocate. Kindness and care were wrapped up together, enveloping Mary and her people. She wanted to care for them and care for her children, protecting them as much as she could from all that their future may hold.

To her children, Grace and Paul, Mary was a hard lady who had had a hard life. Asked to describe her, they revisited times when they were younger and she was firm and distant. A lot had changed as they'd all aged but they still felt the wounds of bitterness and battle-lines long past. Grace and Paul described still working to come to terms with how Mary had treated them, a paired project that seemed to become more urgent as she declined. As Mary slept in her chair, they told me about how they'd spent many hours in the last months sharing memories of their childhood and their parents with each other. Now with children and grandchildren of their own, they'd both only recently begun to feel confident that their parents had loved them as children.

Despite Mary descending into a "cocoon", Grace and Paul felt there were positives about how things were for her now. Mary was "doing well" and was "still there" due to her "spark" and "humour". They also felt that Mary's love for them was now clear. But this welcome understanding was packaged with a near constant need on Mary's part for their reassuring presence, which was an uncomfortably high cost for Grace and Paul.

They also talked about how they'd struggled with the idea of being "completely in charge" of Mary's decisions and her welfare. They'd never been in charge when it came to Mary at any point previously and this new status didn't fit them well. They'd both wanted a way out of being in charge of Mary and they both knew it which made negotiations about who would do what sore and awkward. Surely, they thought, this was a job for a professional, like someone from her healthcare team, a responsible person who could step in easily. Instead, they felt that Mary's clinicians blamed them because Mary had come to hospital "too late". Things had been sliding for Mary for a while. Coming to hospital had become suddenly urgent. Grace and Paul had been made responsible for a decision that should never have been theirs in the first place. They'd been glad that all this seemed to "settle down" with Mary's arrival at the hospice. They seemed relaxed there, finally able to just be with Mary rather than feeling too responsible for what was happening to her.

I met Tom sometime later. Tom seemed tired and careworn, and his kind regard for Mary and her family was clear when he talked about them. He'd been Mary's GP for years and considered himself a witness to all that had changed for her and her family. He spoke a lot about the experience of Mary's kids. Being a carer for a person with dementia was a tough "36 hour a day job" which Tom felt was even more true for Grace and Paul. Mary and her kids had complex relationships, making a tough situation even harder for them. The kids, Grace in particular, felt conflicted about being carers for Mary as they'd never felt that close to her. Tom suspected that this was an unspoken source of tensions between the children, as they both wanted to have a say but neither really wanted to be left in charge. This meant that when things had started going wrong at home, they'd both spent too long looking at each other rather than looking for help.

Tom clearly liked Mary and her family. He'd been involved during good years and bad and ultimately felt he'd shared some of the costs of her decline. He'd found it difficult to notice her deterioration and increasing dependence. He wondered whether knowing them for so long had been helpful or not for Mary and her family. Was his clinical judgement different as a result? He felt that his role was to guide Mary and her family, but he was left feeling unsure how successful he'd been. In Mary's case, he'd felt unsure of how strongly to express his views, as he'd been worried he might have had too strong an influence on her. In the end he felt he'd just stood by, paralysed by familiarity. Briefer relationships with patients could have advantages, noted Tom, observing that it was a nurse meeting Mary at home for the first time who had been able to instigate Mary's admission to the hospice.

System description

In Mary's care network, the relationships and how they had, and hadn't, changed had a potent and complex influence on how this social system worked. Relationships, which were both new and changing while also feeling solid and stable, influenced Mary's communication triggering events that reinforced her sense that it was within her relationships (even very new ones) that her life had value and benefit. Changing relationships influenced Grace's and Paul's memories of their life with their parents now needing to encompass Mary's new needs and relationship with them, and affected how they were able to be with her as children and as carers. This also likely contributed to the difficulty that they expressed around further relationship changes requiring them to feel more responsible for their mother and her welfare. Changing relationships also influenced Tom's expression of the challenges he witnessed within the family and his uncertainty around whether his more established relationship with Mary affected his ability to be her doctor. Within the network, the movement of relationships were interlaced with other sorts of ideas and meanings, like how members identified themselves and each other, and the roles they felt they had or should have within the care system. The changing facets of relationships were powerful and pervasive.

In Mary's network (this social system) the result of all of this influence of the dynamics of relationships seemed to have a number of phases. There was a period of transformation (second-order change) where the system was shaken up by these influences. A new relationship, the home-visiting nurse, was a new component to their care network. Prior to this, the network struggled with how their relationships were changing but without any sense of resolution or progress. The nurse's input and the plan for admission led to a remarkable and previously unavailable series of changes for Mary and everyone. Grace, Paul and Tom all reflected (together and separately) on the reasons for their inability to bring about this change due to their relationships with Mary. Mary had also been able to extend and interpret her sense of meaning within her connection to those around her. While new relationships and further challenges had arisen since that time, the current relationship challenges have resulted in more stable changes (first-order change) within this new context of Mary's being in hospital and hospice. Grace, Paul and Mary in particular now seemed able to explore their responses and communicate with each other through the ongoing changes in relationships without further major changes to the care system occurring. In system terms, the ongoing influence of this relationship work was now resulting in stable changes in the system where the form and function of their social system seemed to be maintained.

Other examples of the impacts of the shifts and movement of relationships were evident for other care networks. The dynamics of longer-term relationships, such as new difficulties or sustained difficulties which now faced new pressures and unfamiliar contexts, or how old relationships meant different things over time with qualities lost or gained, all had an impact on how social systems changed and moved. Similarly, new relationships and what they could bring, disturb, create and draw attention to had a profound impact. Changing relationships were frequent sources of influence in dementia care networks.

Power and status

Dementia often seems to change who within a care network seems to have the power and what kinds of power they have. These sorts of dynamics can have potent effects on how the care network shifts and moves under the influence of these changes in status. For some dementia care networks, these dynamics seemed to be influential when there was a change in focus about who the system was "for". Care networks could respond to these influences with significant transformations in how the care network functioned. Triggers for this sort of shift often seemed to be a change in the network to now focus more on the needs of a person with dementia due to their progressing issues. Counter-intuitively, there could also be similar changes in the network's focus with progression of dementia toward the carer and away from the person with dementia. Power dynamics could also influence the network when new ways of understanding and making sense of the shifts in power and status had taken place. These seemed to trigger more stable and less dramatic changes in how the networks worked when these occurred. The following story from Ken's care network will explore how power and status changes influenced his network.

Ken's care network's story

Meeting Ken for the first time, the word "bookish" sprang to mind. I think he'd have had good odds at being accurately picked out as an academic within any line-up. Ken and Sarah were charming, kind, well-read people who'd married, raised a family and lived together in a comfortable home in a nice suburb.

Ken saw his life as a success story. He'd been a well-regarded academic in Australia and abroad who'd made a significant contribution in his area of expertise of social work and social studies. He'd been drawn to his work from a young age. His memory of this time in the UK was one of vast social upheaval and uncertainty which had left many people insecure and unsupported. Witnessing this happening all around him, he'd wanted to be able to do something worthwhile and positive, to do his bit to help the many people who needed it. Maybe it was also his own challenges that had drawn him to the plight of others. Ken was born with a progressing eye problem which meant he had always been visually impaired and had needed a lot of surgeries and other healthcare input. His determination to help others seemed only matched by his refusal to have his life dictated by his own, lifelong health challenges.

He felt he'd needed patience and a steadfast attitude to manage, and this seemed clearly in evidence in all that he'd put his hand to.

Ken's take on life was that it presented a series of opportunities to grow and understand. He felt that this perspective had helped him become a "big noise" professionally but had also helped him realise when that phase of his life had passed. Walking away from his career, though, had been so much easier to reconcile than being told that he had dementia. Ken felt he understood deeply the frailties of ageing and just didn't think this label "dementia" fit him. He didn't think it applied and was certain it wasn't helpful. Ken suspected that diagnosing dementia was a "fad" for doctors, and they probably threw that term around too much. He also thought that his visual impairment probably made assessing him more complicated and wasn't sure they'd properly taken that into account. Ken felt that being told he had "dementia" made him feel less certain of himself and less trusting of his own perceptions. The dementia label hadn't explained anything for Ken, he felt it had just harmed him further. Overall, Ken felt that given that he'd spent a lifetime successfully coping with one major health problem, a new diagnosis like dementia didn't seem fair.

Sarah's view on all of this was a little different. She hadn't been shocked or even surprised when Ken had been diagnosed with dementia. Sarah's memory was that Ken had been worried about his cognition for years prior to his assessment in the memory clinic. She'd walked into that room fully anticipating the results that they'd been told. She thought that may have been why she felt so prepared for each step of what had happened since. Ken refused to feel threatened by his dementia. Sarah's own take on it, however, was that it's hard to predict what will happen next for any of us. But Sarah had her suspicions when it came to Ken's future. She'd worked as a nurse for many years and felt clear about where his future was heading. Sarah said she didn't want to think about this and, consequently, she and Ken didn't talk about his dementia at all. They'd rarely discussed it with anyone. A few years earlier, they had revealed the diagnosis to their friends. Sarah thought this was important to do to avoid future isolation and embarrassment, and Ken went along with it.

Coping, for Sarah, was a matter of preparation. She'd always organised and approached Ken's dementia by leaning on these same strengths. Her planning hadn't led them astray thus far, and she felt hopeful that they'd negotiate their way through what was happening now. Ken's ability to cope despite all the health issues he had was admittedly central to her plan. Sarah felt it was important to let him continue to test himself, even if it was clearly risky now. Sarah wasn't sure it was an easy balance to get right, and their wedding anniversary party reminded Sarah that she wasn't always the best judge of what was manageable for him. Ken had always been a skilled orator and Sarah didn't think much about asking him, as always, to give a speech at their party. After the night's glow had faded, she realised that he'd worked unusually hard to "live up to" his usual standards. Belatedly, Sarah understood that now more than ever, Ken was worried about disappointing her. And Sarah did need Ken to continue to work hard. Their relationship had always worked through her being able to get her space when she needed it, and she needed that now. Sarah had a three-week trip away coming up. She thought Ken would manage by himself but they hadn't talked much about this, at least in part because he would have to manage. When does coping with and ignoring dementia actually become its own kind of burden, Sarah wondered.

Jade was a specialist geriatrician who'd become involved in Ken's care as the specialist who'd given him his diagnosis of dementia. Her role in Ken's and Sarah's care felt typical for her. She felt that her main role was to provide a diagnosis for her patients and that was what she'd done for Ken. Jade loved to diagnose problems. It was neat and satisfying. For her, it also made her job interesting, challenging and important. The decision about what was going on was hers alone. While she worked in a team, Jade felt that she was "the captain" due to the responsibility to decide and declare what everyone should think about what was happening. Jade was deeply satisfied with the work she did, and felt that others, particularly patients and their families, were satisfied too.

Jade felt her input into Sarah's and Ken's lives had been typical. She also felt that they were "good" patients, accepting the diagnosis "gracefully" and coping well with what had happened. This wasn't a surprise. Jade believed that the community as a whole was now coping better with dementia and that people now hoped and believed that dementia is another "treatable" condition. Jade explained that she didn't think that dementia had become more treatable. But she did feel that fostering this hope in others was one of her professional roles. Not telling the whole truth about dementia was, from Jade's perspective, an important aspect of the care that she was tasked with providing.

Jade felt that she understood why Sarah and Ken had told me that she was their dementia doctor, but she felt differently. From her perspective, her relationship with them was largely over, confined to that critical role of providing a diagnosis. She didn't feel particularly connected to them now. As with all her patients, her involvement was not prolonged. She'd met and assessed them, made a decision, and then they'd left her life.

System description

In Ken's network, the dominant influence on how the system worked seemed to relate to the dynamics of power and status of network members. Ken's independent and highly regarded status — maintained despite the adversity of his health conditions — was challenged by the dementia diagnosis. His response was to distrust and ignore the relevance of this new unhelpful label. Jade perceived herself as the minimally involved "captain" of the ship who chose what to reveal to others about their illness and who highlighted how manageable it was. This sat in tension with the resistance Ken and Sarah had to their lives being dictated to by dementia. At the same time, Sarah struggled with her own professional insight as a nurse (knowing that Ken would get worse) and her uncertain role in supporting his increasingly risky independence which she felt she relied upon. Sarah had a significant degree of power within their relationship as an organiser and primary voice in what they would do, but Ken's needs were unwelcome challenges to this dynamic. Similarly, their need for the support of others like Jade felt similarly unfamiliar and uncomfortable, made more so by Jade's strict and powerful determination that she was no longer available for them.

Ken's diagnosis of dementia has challenged the dementia system in terms of these important dynamics of status and power. These challenges seemed largely to lead to stable change responses (first-order change) where significant changes in the way the system functioned hadn't occurred. This was due to these challenges being interpreted and responded to by the system using pre-existing types of communication and meanings that the care system had available to it, like Ken's independent identity and Sarah's role in determining how they will cope with what's occurring. However, Sarah's reflections on her own contribution to these difficulties within the story, and the potential need for more attention to dementia seemed to hint at the potential for further system perturbations related to status and power. If Sarah's reflections result in her adopting a more powerful position within the network to focus on these issues, or if Ken's responses to his changing cognition shift, it's foreseeable that more transformative changes in the care system may result.

How we are individually

The types of influences on care systems we've discussed so far all relate to influences on the bonds and links between people, how they were together. But changes and influences on a more individual level could also lead to detectable movement in the system as a whole. The primary cause for this often seemed to involve the impact of identity and selfhood, and how these were seen as challenged, changed, compromised or continuing.

Identity and selfhood

Identity and selfhood, particularly when changed or challenged, was a significant and frequent perturbing influence in care systems in my study. In some care systems, for instance, this occurred when people continued to assert identities which no longer seemed to fit the system's expectations. These challenges also seemed to arise when there were significant changes in people with dementia's personalities or what they seemed to value. Some care systems also expressed this kind of influence when it became uncertain whether people with dementia could continue to have an identity due to their advancing condition and changes to communication. The responding changes in the care networks resulting from these challenges could be radical. When people were no longer seen as "themselves", network changes which redefined what care meant and how it should be provided were common. More subtle stabilising changes could also result under the influence of movements of identity when changes in how selves were expressed or how identity was recognised involved new, but accessible, types of communication. Nicholas's care network story provides an example of some of the changes and responses.

Nicholas's care network's story

Nicholas had his story all mapped out. He stepped me through it as we sat in armchairs in his living room. Nicholas was a thinker and a man of logic. He viewed his working life as a clear progression of successful outcomes, all related to his ability to rationally solve problems using the scientific method. His achievements had been exceptional. He had been a "pioneer" who had been able to overcome novel challenges and succeed where others had not due to his character and his capacity.

Nicholas's confidence in science was total. Others with whom he disagreed were often viewed as not being "scientific". Nicholas felt that such disagreements wouldn't happen if others had his insight. The real answers were obvious viewed in the right way. Nicholas felt it was only natural that he would extend his successful approach to life to his diagnosis of dementia. He saw himself as "new" to dementia. Even if he'd had the diagnosis for some time, it was an experience he was still getting to know, to understand and to adapt to. One understanding that Nicholas had come to was that dementia could have a negative effect on him, but he hadn't experienced this. He was confidently hopeful he never would. For someone like him, dementia was a problem that could be overcome. Nicholas was happy that he remained active, involved and supportive at home with Hanna, his wife, and continued to enjoy the exercise and activities that he participated in around town.

Hanna was fairly quiet sitting with us while Nicholas shared his story, waiting for a private moment at another time to provide a different telling. Nicholas had always been a "nice man" overall from Hanna's perspective, but he hadn't been the peerless success he remembered. He'd struggled as a husband and father and had been difficult to deal with. His relationship with Hanna and with the kids had always been troubled. Work was also more of a challenge for him than he now recalled. He'd changed jobs a lot, always being quiet about why, but Hanna felt that he'd not really fit in with his workmates either. She'd never needed more explanation than that though. She felt she'd always understood his difficulties back then, even if he'd never shared them.

Hanna knew that Nicholas was working as hard as he could to cope with what was happening to them because of his dementia, but she felt that his struggling and thrashing against it was slowly dragging her under. He was fixated on "taking control" of his dementia through busy work of planning and organising. She'd realised, over time, that he couldn't see that his efforts made no sense. Hanna confessed that she found his preoccupations pathetic, small ideas from a fading man, but also felt guilty for this as it was clearly important to him. They disagreed frequently on a host of topics but Hanna felt too tired to be bothered fighting with him anymore. The stage of their lives involving her trying to convince him of anything had well and truly passed. He didn't listen and couldn't change. Now Hannah noticed that she just left him out of most of their decisions, even the ones relating to his dementia. It was just easier that way, and she didn't have the energy for anything difficult.

In her own way, Hanna knew that she was also engaged in her own torpid fight to cope. She had plenty of offers of help, but nothing made things easier for her. She didn't need support to be a carer, she wanted opportunities to allow her to be something or someone else. The little energy she had left was reserved for escape. She wondered if part of what she wanted to run from was the imagined "awful silence" when Nicholas was no longer there. She could feel it and her grief coming toward her.

Stewart had been working in this area and caring for this community for over 30 years. He lived around the corner from Hanna and Nicholas and knew a lot of his patients from around town. Nicholas was no exception. They'd known each other before he'd become his GP, and he'd been his GP for decades. One thing that Stewart was sure of was that Nicholas was different. He was now a "shell of his old self", simultaneously the same and a completely different person due to his dementia. "How do you doctor in dementia?" Stewart mused. Stewart wasn't sure what to make of the "issues" that Nicholas brought into his clinic. Hanna would often describe physical symptoms but Nicholas wouldn't remember having them. "Whose problem are they then?", Stewart wondered. Over time Stewart had determined that the best way of dealing with Nicholas's unremembered problems was to ignore them.

Stewart felt more comfortable with his role in helping Nicholas and Hanna face challenges as they arose. Thinking and planning for the future was another matter. There hadn't been a right time yet, from his side of the desk. Stewart felt that they were probably in denial. In his experience, families weren't often prepared to "grasp the nettle". Planning for the future with dementia meant planning and making changes, both of which were often resisted by the person with the diagnosis. It was a tough ask to do what was necessary, and he wasn't sure that Hanna was up to it. Stewart felt that she had planned well for now and he wasn't sure that she would be able to do so for what would come later. In many ways, Stewart felt, it would be easier to manage these sorts of problems if clinicians with the necessary experience could just explain and insist on the right solution when they perceived that there was one.

System description

Identity was highly influential in Nicholas's care network, particularly ripples from Nicholas's asserting a strong and unchanged sense of his own identity and Hanna's reluctant self-empowerment. Nicholas saw himself as growing through dementia to become more of the man he already felt he was. For Nicholas, overcoming dementia was an extension of who he was within the powerful "truth" of his "scientific method", factors which were both of persisting and growing relevance for Nicholas as explanations for why he was different from his apparent story. Hanna perceived Nicholas's expressed identity as a pathetic fraud. The further he moved from this version of himself the tighter his focus on it became. She resigned herself to drifting apart from the new and increasingly problematic version of Nicholas even as she grieved him. Hanna wearily embraced a new view of herself in response to Nicholas's changes, someone who was more in control of their shared life than she had ever been before. Stewart struggled to identify who Nicholas was now and devalued his dementia-affected experiences. Stewart interpreted Nicholas's and Hanna's difficulties as their own failure and believed that they had made things worse by not allowing him to tell them what they should do, even though he, also, didn't seem clear what changes were needed. Together, the shifting challenge of Nicholas's and Hanna's identity changes had been responded to by transformation (second-order change) within this care system at this point in their story. While care remained a focus, the idea of what that meant and who it was for had become nebulous and unclear for this network. The shifts of Nicholas's and Hanna's identities had led to communication which tended to work around and against other network members rather than through collaboration. Nicholas's identity no longer seemed to include a story other than his own. Hanna's increasing identity as the decision-maker wasn't arrived at through growth but rather because there were no other options and drastic changes were needed. Her reflections about the difficulties of working with Nicholas's past identity throughout their lives seemed to imply a long period of stability, of making things work throughout their relationship together. The impact of dementia on the network and specifically on Nicholas's identity, however, meant that those previous stabilising responses to changes just weren't enough anymore.

Changes within individuals' identities and experience of selfhood had a significant impact on dementia networks leading to multiple and sometimes drastic responses from those networks.

Our perception

Dementia care systems also seemed to be influenced by the direct experience of dementia changes themselves. This seemed distinct from the previous types of influence discussed, as these experiences weren't changes that were perceived as being changes within the people in the network (how we are individually), or how those people connected with each other (how we are together) but were more directly appreciated as being because of the dementia itself. This sort of influence wasn't specifically understood as being about people but about dementia's influence on daily experiences, the anticipation of events, how past events were now interpreted, and how the meanings associated with these perceptions had an impact on care systems and led them to respond to these changes. In the stories and their descriptions below the primary catalyst for these influences is, unsurprisingly, the changes associated with dementia itself. Other triggers, including changes in care associated with being in hospital or residential care, the perception of suffering, or anticipation of behavioural disturbance and aggression, could all potentially contribute to similar challenges for systems.

Today's experiences

The experience of the present, what days felt like and what they included, was often a source of challenge and change for care networks. The challenges and influences of daily experiences usually involved dementia symptoms, like memory loss or communication changes, and what these were felt to mean. These changes and challenges could have significant impacts on how these care networks worked and functioned. Small stable changes of doing things differently, "working around the dementia", where the network didn't undergo major shifts were common. Larger transformations with major implications for the structure of the care network, such as through a person with dementia moving to a care facility to live, could also be system responses.

Interestingly, but not surprisingly, there also seemed to be connections between these sorts of challenges and the types we've already discussed, as changes in daily experiences could lead to changes in how people were individually and how they were together.

Ronald's care network's story

Ronald had always been someone who'd been listened to. He'd been a Christian minister who had led his flock for many years. He was wise and well-read. He'd always had a sense of confidence about how things were and how they should be. However, there seemed no doubt in his mind that things had changed. Ever since he'd been diagnosed with dementia it had all been different. He now felt that his perspectives and recollections were discounted, passed over, unreliable. It was as if something about his ability to read the world had shifted for everyone but him. And it all seemed to be getting worse.

My meeting him seemed symbolic of this hard-to-define change. Here I was, a total stranger, in his house asking him about dementia. Something significant had obviously changed but he wasn't quite sure what, or why? I asked him about memory loss and Ronald responded with his own questions. He wondered about what losing your memory means. What does it mean to lose something so insubstantial? Ronald himself wasn't aware of forgetting things even though others assured that he did. So, who's problem was that really? Seeing the poise in his steady gaze at me, I was quite sure who's problem Ronald felt it was.

Ronald's tone invited disagreement. He told me he understood, of course, that he might be unaware that he had forgotten things, but that it still seemed to him that his perspective should be seen as the most valid one. He could live much more freely than others gave him credit for but felt that his potential for contribution and independence was ignored. Ronald rejected the sense that he was diminished by his dementia. He joked, with a vague but apparent edge, that he lived a secret life when his wife wasn't home, his eyes again holding a challenge to suggest otherwise. Of course, a lot had changed since his diagnosis, Ronald acknowledged, but the dementia hadn't forced any specific changes upon him. He'd made a variety of difficult, but ultimately timely, "right" choices after his diagnosis. He had decided to retire from his church ministry and to give up his driver's licence because he'd reasoned it through and got it "right". That left him now with less to do but a lot to enjoy. His time at home post-retirement didn't "drag".

He took pride in the small chores he did at home. Ronald expressed how the most important parts of his life had not changed at all, such as his faith in God and his enjoyment of sharing his life with his wife. But while treasured, these experiences were still difficult to talk about. Asked for details, Ronald often seemed to be unable to find the answers he expected and clearly found that frustrating and inexplicable.

Jenny didn't say much when I was talking to Ronald. Later, she expressed a different but important other side to their story that she felt needed to be heard. She also struggled to be able to put what Ronald's dementia meant for them into words, not because it was ephemeral, but so present and central that it was difficult to get a vantage point from which to describe it. It had, simply, affected everything, every aspect of their life. It was a pervasive larceny where nothing was secure enough or sacred enough to be safe. The most wounding part of this for Jenny was that dementia had robbed them of their partnership.

They'd had their fair share of challenges but had always overcome things together. But now, they were just drifting away from each other in their "going through the motions", enabling just enough of who they had been for each other to get by. Jenny was reminded of F. Scott Fitzgerald's Gatsby staring across the bay and felt they were similarly "beating on against the current day by day", committed to a "dreary" and tragic effort. Jenny described her efforts to engage Ronald in their life but seemed exhausted even by talking about it. The process required to meaningfully involve him was taking everything that she had left, and she struggled to keep trying. Now, feeling like she was facing the enormity of what was happening alone felt unfair, sad and lonely. Sometimes it was way too much and Jenny felt like just screaming, but she wasn't even sure she'd have the energy to make a noise. It would just be her distressed face, like in the painting by Munch, silently calling out in pain. Previously, her faith had been a solace. But like so much of their lives this had been a shared resource too and it all felt so much "dimmer" to Jenny now. Sometimes, she got frustrated with him and his ignorance of what was happening. Once, she'd noticed with some degree of shame and horror that she was starting to talk to him in the teacher's voice that she used to use to scold her pupils from many years ago. Ronald had become someone she needed to manage, rather than her partner.

But she was glad that Ronald didn't seem to appreciate that loss or the mounting toll for which his dementia was responsible. With a teary smile she said that she did wish that he would grieve a little more, grieve losing her as he was losing himself. Or that she felt that it would be lovely if, at the very least, he'd notice how hard she was working and how she never did anything for herself anymore. But she felt that it was her pain to bear. Jenny was reconciled to being lonely in grief and fighting for the life they'd had together. There didn't seem to be any real help for her. Jenny even found (GP) Chris's care unsatisfying. Ronald seemed to like him, perhaps, she wondered, because he never really asked them any meaningful questions about how they were going. That probably meant that Ronald never felt threatened by him. Jenny, though, felt that his only interest seemed to be in writing new scripts. He certainly didn't seem to be that interested in how she was coping.

Chris had been Ronald's GP for many years. We spoke with each other over the phone and Chris went through what had occurred with a matter-of-fact air. It was Jenny who'd first noticed that Ronald's memory seemed to be changing. She'd prompted Chris to look further into this, which he'd done. The results had confirmed that there was a problem. Chris felt that Ronald had "taken this in stride" and decided that he needed to step away from his work as a minister. As he reflected, though, Chris noted that he wasn't sure how Ronald felt about his condition or his situation now. They hadn't really talked about anything like that recently. Chris described a "hunch" that Ronald might "need to feel relevant" but he hadn't asked him about it. It wasn't clear that any of these questions were going to be resolved soon. Chris didn't feel that there would be much sense in "drilling down" into how Ronald was feeling about these kinds of issues. He described his sense that Ronald's "understanding and insight" were too limited for it to be worthwhile to discuss these kinds of issues.

On the other hand, Chris believed that Jenny was very able. He wondered if this might be its own kind of problem. Chris mused that Jenny wished to have an active and involved life which made things harder for both of them as Ronald couldn't and didn't want to be involved. The solution, from Chris's perspective, was for Jenny to decide that it was time for Ronald to move to a care facility. This would make it much easier for her to have the life she wanted. He suspected that she'd been thinking about this for a while and that Ronald's last day at home would be soon. Chris didn't feel he had much he could offer them. Short GP consultations didn't allow for much that felt meaningful in this situation. But still, seeing him did allow Jenny somewhere that was safe for her to voice her worries and concerns, and that was something.

System description

In Ronald's story we can see that "today's experience" of dementia seemed to have a big impact on the care system and how it responded. Dementia didn't have a specific meaning for Ronald. He experienced it as an unclear absence with the irritating characteristic of making others regard him as diminished. His stern defence against this, expressing that he remained unchanged and largely unaffected by his dementia, left little space for alternative perspectives to be explored. Chris, on the other hand, saw dementia as indicating that Ronald wasn't really a contributor to the network anymore. For Chris, the dementia experience meant that Ronald had become a complication which had a negative impact on Jenny's life and her choices. Dementia meant that Chris didn't really see himself as caring for Ronald anymore, his role had changed to someone who continued to see them partly because there weren't alternatives to his being involved, and partly to support Jenny to have somewhere to say how hard it was living with Ronald. Jenny struggled to express how significant dementia was for Ronald and her. The change for her was profound. Dementia meant that she'd not only lost much of what was important to her through the loss of mutual interests but also how she found value in those important experiences because so much of that came through sharing them with Ronald. This experience touched and changed everything and her lifelong way of making sense of challenges, working them through with Ronald, was an option also lost to her.

The current dementia experience the network was faced with caused problems but also disrupted the usual tools to respond to them within the network. These experiences of dementia influenced the network, diminishing the possibility of communication and the willingness of the people involved in the system to continue to try to connect. Responses within the network were transformative but didn't seem to be associated with growth or resilience. Rather, the changes taking place seemed to suggest disengagement and disconnection, particularly in respect to diminishment of the close partnership that Jenny and Ronald had shared prior to dementia's impact. For this network, the idea of "care" had dissolved into uncertainty and distance. Further significant changes to the network, with the potential for a need for additional supports or (as Chris felt was required) consideration of Ronald moving to residential care all seemed possible given the challenges the care system was responding to. It was also clear that other perturbations such as relationship and identity changes could be important influences on this care network now and into the future.

The future

Dementia experiences aren't always only felt in the present. These experiences also often seemed to mean something for how care networks thought, talked and acted relative to what they felt their future was now going to be like. In this way, dementia's impact on anticipated future experiences was common and had a powerful influence on how dementia networks responded to the changes taking place. The sorts of futures which seemed to influence networks included perceptions of future high degrees of dependence, diminished communication or recognition of network members and family, a need for moving to an aged care facility, or dying from dementia. What the future might mean or hold for care systems could result in either dramatic changes for networks if the anticipated future was felt to be outside of what the system could support, or more stable changes if this seemed within what the system could communicate through and work with.

Frank's network's story

Frank was a kindly looking man with a quick smile and an easy laugh. He had recently moved into an upstairs apartment in a supported accommodation facility with his wife, Julie, which was where I met them both. I was struck by a number of colourfully decorated, hand-bound books and when I asked about them Julie told me that Frank had made them. Frank told me that they were books of memories. Conscious of his fallible memory, Frank had started documenting what he wanted to remember. This had started with notes to himself but had ended up being something with deeper meaning. Frank realised that others might also be interested in reading his memories stored in writing, and so he started documenting and delicately illustrating his own life-stories as a legacy to leave for his children and grandkids. Each of Frank's stories was a little chapter that spoke about the "good" that he felt he'd done, what he felt that meant and why that was important. They were like little fables that guided his family towards how Frank saw the world. Frank believed that he had a life that was "worth remembering" and he hoped that the books captured the spirit of that.

Writing things down as a response to memory loss expressed the calm sensibility that Frank extended to all the challenges of his dementia. He felt that it was important to "cope" and "make do" regardless of life's challenges, and dementia was no different. Frank did feel that his life had changed due to his diagnosis but "not uncomfortably" so. For Frank, he was now living a "life of retracted things" where he "walk(ed) down familiar roads", but that in itself wasn't that important to him. More important to Frank was how he lived the life that he had now.

Frank felt that his spirituality deeply affected who he was. He understood his future through his faith and his mission to bring others closer to his God. He didn't think his faith had been limited by dementia. Maybe how he expressed his faith had but the depth of it hadn't and for Frank this made his future feel comfortable and reassuring. If anything, Frank felt that dementia had made him feel more fully aware of his relationship to his God, something that Frank was genuinely thankful for. The idea of a future where he died of dementia wasn't scary as it was just a step towards an afterlife with his God about which he felt vividly confident. Dementia, on some levels, had given him more than it had taken away.

Julie shared Frank's life and his beliefs but didn't and couldn't feel the same way. She wanted to experience and maintain Frank's conviction but it was always out of reach. Dementia, again and again, stood in the way of her feeling balanced and in control. She wished for the equanimity that Frank seemed effortlessly to maintain in the face of dementia. But she felt she quaked and struggled to cope as a carer. It was all stressful and frustrating. She tried to remind herself that when she got irritated it was with Frank's dementia, and not with Frank. He didn't seem to mind though, and she mostly loved him for that. In many ways, she felt their love for each other was clearer than ever before, even if there were also more hidden difficulties.

For Julie, their future was threatening and uncertain. There were too many unknowns and too much certainty that she would have to figure everything out and make it work. Julie felt most comfortable being practical and "getting things right". She wanted to plan for what might come but didn't know what to do with this drive given that planning was so difficult. Julie knew that Frank would accept anything she suggested was needed to make things easier. She'd felt that moving into supported accommodation would make her feel more confident, and Frank had been happy to do that. He'd done it for her even though he'd loved their home. Frank wanted to help but Julie believed that he had little insight into the things that concerned her. A big worry for her was that Frank's decline might be slow and prolonged, and more than she was able to manage even with the change to the apartment. Living next to the local nursing home was a frequent and unpalatable reminder of a future that Julie feared for both of their sakes. Frank, of course, didn't seem that worried, but Julie openly hoped that he would die soon to avoid all of that happening. She hoped that their faith was enough to sustain them until then.

Tony had only recently become Frank's and Julie's GP, even though he had known them for years. They had been members of the same Christian congregation for a long time. Not that long ago, Frank and Julie had asked him to take on this additional role as their doctor. Tony had agreed and felt that the transition in their relationships together had been relatively easy. But there was also no doubt that he couldn't be the same friend and community member for them now as he had been in the past. Tony felt that he could no longer be anything other than their doctor and, so, no longer considered them as anything other than his patients.

Tony felt that his strongest connection to the couple was through Julie. He was conscious of carefully trying to parcel out information to Julie, to prepare her for the future with Frank that he felt was coming. This required some thought and delicacy for Tony. He rationed what he told her about his forecasting of their future. Tony worried that revealing too much, explaining how difficult he thought it would actually be, would unfairly burden Julie. Tony felt that it was inevitable that Frank would require care in a facility. He was very confident that Frank's care needs would eclipse what Julie might be able to support or plan for at home. He hadn't discussed this with them either. He didn't feel that this kind of information was relevant for them, given they seemed happy and hopeful in their new apartment.

Tony felt that his role as Frank's and Julie's doctor was to provide support. On the other hand, he also felt that most of what he was able to offer was to stay involved and to observe what happened. For Tony, conditions like dementia were representative of humanity's imperfection. As flawed creations, there is no way we can escape our fate. The only option available is the necessary personal journal of coming to terms with the lot that is given to us. Seen like this, Tony felt that Frank's dementia and his unavoidable future decline was an opportunity for learning for everyone. He suspected that the lesson for Julie would be about the limits of her faith. She was trying to balance her faith, her commitment to her husband, and her own needs. He wasn't sure that she'd be able to keep it all stable, but he knew that trying would consume a lot of energy. Tony believed that Julie's inability to accept the advice he'd given about Frank's illness and her worry about the future made clear that she was having difficulty coming to terms with what would happen.

System description

The influence of the anticipated future with dementia was powerful in Ken's care network. Frank's sense of his future was reassuring. It tied in with a view of his life as a complete and virtuous story to be handed on. It echoed his conviction in his faith and his view that his illness and dying were a transition to better things. Frank saw his future with dementia as a transcendence which would be beneficial for him, and instructive for others. Dementia was not the sole cause of this deeper transformation for Frank, but it played a clear part in influencing what his future meant to him. Julie's approach to her future was tied closely to her awareness that her relationship with Frank was changing and that these changes would continue. She couldn't feel Frank's sense of faith that their future was a good one. She worried at her inability to plan and prepare and feared for the future that she felt Frank's dementia was likely to bring to them. She openly hoped that he would die early to prevent an experience she was confident was not what she wanted. Tony believed that the challenges of the future required everyone within the care network to learn and grow. Because Frank had dementia and because he was an imperfect human, Tony knew that he was bound to need more help than Julie could provide, but learning this might be an unfair burden. More useful would be for them all to develop their faith. Tony privately believed that he had already achieved the growth that the other network members needed, and that Julie's primary struggle was with her own lack of faith.

We can see that the challenges of the future led to a transformation within this care network. There were different and competing interpretations within the care network about what the future entailed and how to respond to it. What faith meant to network members and how this related to how Frank's health might decline seemed central to how the shared future of the network was understood and related to. These influences resulted in a transformation in how caring was understood and discussed within the network. Understanding what Frank's decline might look like and how the network would respond to it didn't have simple, uniform answers although the relationship of ideas of faith to these differences seemed clearer. The response within the network was a change in communication. There was less shared understanding or exploration of these differences in perspective about the future and what that meant for the network. It remains to be seen whether these challenges could be reconciled but the current focus on faith with its different meanings for network members as a way of explaining Frank's future and its impact on those around him seemed unlikely to lead to an improvement in the cohesion of this care network.

4. Making sense of change

These stories have come from real moments in the lives of real people. I've tried to frame them in a way that shares with you something about how I think dementia care networks seem to change and react in response to the challenges that come up in dementia. I hope that I've gone some way to convince you of that idea — that dementia care networks are influenced by the sorts of challenges that dementia throws at them, and that these challenges and how the networks respond are central to what we experience as "dementia".

Maybe you're willing to meet me at that point. Perhaps it's true that these changes happen, but is it important? Again, I think that it almost couldn't be more important. What this tells us is that listening to the stories of dementia care networks can help us detect not just what is influencing them, what's rocking the boat so to speak, but where that's leaving them. Is this new wave of change that is welling up from new challenges in relationships or how a person with dementia sees themselves helping them balance the boat? Is it water-tight or spilling the network and leaving them floundering?

I think that these sorts of stories show us that if we're paying the right kind of attention, listening to a network rather than just a person, we can detect the sorts of influences that challenge and perturb dementia care systems. I'd also suggest that we've been able to describe a sense of a "dominant" perturbation in each of these stories which made sense within the story and helped describe the kinds of change that seemed to be detectable within the care networks. On many levels, we shouldn't feel surprised by this. If we accept the notions of systems theory and social systems, care networks do function as small care systems and will be influenced or perturbed by different factors. The challenge that we've tried to respond to here was to detect these influences and make them apparent.

I should also note, however, that there is much that has been simplified in making these observations and judgments. Systems have been described as happening "all at once" and connected in "many directions simultaneously" (Meadows, 2008: 253). Identifying the influences affecting networks in these stories and describing them as "dominant" hopefully makes sense in the context of what's happening in these stories. But that doesn't mean that these influences are the only things affecting these care networks. It also doesn't mean that these influences *remained* the most important things affecting these networks. The stories take place within a particular time reflecting the time that I was involved in the lives of these people. What happened after that might indicate that something else entirely was going on and affecting the care network. As I've tried to make clear, the stories we have discussed highlight that engaging with those systems at different times might have revealed different important influences or that different types of change responses were taking place. It's also possible that there are other important influences than the three broad groups that we've identified in this work, and that the work here hasn't captured everything. It's reasonable for us to be a bit cautious in assuming that what is evident is automatically significant or represents the entirety of something. Like the blind man describing an elephant while he's holding its tail, there may be a lot left for us to discover. What we have to work with from these stories doesn't offer us a complete answer to understanding dementia care systems, but it does reveal more than would have been obvious otherwise.

For instance, the three core groups of influences that were important in these stories: "how we are together", "how we are individually" and "our perception" seem to make some intuitive sense. These fit well with the themes and issues that people with dementia, their family carers and their paid carers tended to want and need to talk about (in Part Two of this book). From what we've explored together dementia seems quite commonly to lead to questions and challenges related to who we are alone and together and how we make sense of our experiences. Many of the ripples dementia causes in care networks would be able to be related back to these groups. If that seems like a reasonable enough conclusion, we're starting to get close to an even more important step. If we can define a useful framework that can be used to help detect and identify the sorts of challenges that occur within dementia networks, we are on threshold of being able to do something about it when we need to.

Having reached this understanding, we might now want to anticipate what comes next for the dementia care system. Mary's story, for instance, included events and influences which indicated a transition from an unstable, transformative response in the care system — relating to the relationships and corresponding to the mounting challenges at home and the need for new relationships to provide the best care — to a more stable phase. This stability was achieved by new relationships and new approaches to relationships brought about by this transformation. This sort of pattern is frequently observed in systems. Major transformation (second-order changes) within social systems can be required for systems to become more stable and more resilient to future challenges (Bateson, 1972a). For Mary's network, the move to the hospital was a major shake-up for their care network but, ultimately, that environment, and the space to reflect and re-define what they all felt for each other without needing the kids to be "carers", allowed things to settle into a new type of comfortable equilibrium. I'd say this was despite the dementia but, truthfully, it happened because of the dementia. Not the dementia alone, mind you, but the changes rippling out from the dementia were central to the responses that led to all of this eventually occurring.

Major transformations aren't always good for systems, though. If in Mary's network the initial transformation had been followed by still more periods of upheaval, it's probable that the comfortable stability that we described would have been elusive. Stabilising responses (minor adjustments without major upheaval — also called first order change) also aren't always good for systems. If a ship is sailing into an iceberg, a small course correction might not cut it. Like refusing to say sorry because the other person hasn't either, sometimes staying the course can lead to disaster. Stabilising responses at the wrong moment can lead to systems deteriorating or dissolving (Meadows, 2008). If we think about the living system of a growing sapling that lives in poor soil, my providing it with fertiliser and improving the soil quality may lead to a transformation of that tree's living system, ultimately leading to its growth and further stability. Allowing the stable systemic processes of the tree to continue to do its best with the poor soil may eventually lead to the tree dying. However, context is important. Adding fertiliser if the season is wrong or if the tree is too dry may also be transformative but in a way which leads to the tree dying. Likewise, leaving a flourishing tree to continue its stable changes in response to its environment may be the best chance that it has to continue to flourish. Whether transformative or stabilising, change states are "good" or "bad" for the system depending on what else seems to be occurring.

Being able to assess what seems to be perturbing a dementia care system, and whether this seems to be leading to stable or transformative changes potentially enables us to anticipate what might happen next in the context of that system. The concepts of system resilience and vulnerability are useful to support thinking this through. Resilience and vulnerability relate to a system's capacity to withstand shocks, surprises and unforeseen or hazardous circumstances, and its access to the resources it requires to meet these challenges (Langridge & Christian-Smith, 2006). Resilience and vulnerability therefore affect the potential for, and the response to, perturbation and change states within care systems and have implications for their ability to continue to achieve their function of maintaining care and support. I'd suggest that, in Mary's story above, the transformation we explored together meant that their system was more resilient. It was more prepared for what was happening to all of them and, crucially, what was happening to Mary. Having resilient care systems in dementia seems an important goal. As we've discussed, dementia is a progressive condition and never ceases raising new challenges and problems. Resilient care systems would be as well-prepared for whatever the new challenge might be as they can be, better able to support each other to crest the waves. If we can understand and detect what perturbs or influences the dementia care system (of people) in front of us, we are taking a first step towards knowing whether what's happening might lead to that care system becoming more resilient or more vulnerable.

Rippling out and bouncing back

As we've noted, people with dementia and those who care for them face many challenges. Being able to anticipate what might make these care systems more vulnerable or more resilient is an important idea. However, the implications and potential in detecting and understanding the factors that influence care systems goes deeper. Within the dementia care network stories that we shared it was clear that changes in an individual person associated with dementia (that is, changes within the various mental, communicative and physical systems which make up that person) lead to influences on the social systems surrounding them. These system changes ripple outward from dementia's impact. But the ripples don't only move in one direction. As we discussed earlier, Kitwood and others have also told us that the personal experience of dementia is influenced by broader factors like how communities and societies engage with dementia. One of Kitwood's examples, you may remember, was that what people think about people with dementia tends to create that reality. If we see people with dementia as unable to be involved in society, that, ultimately, is

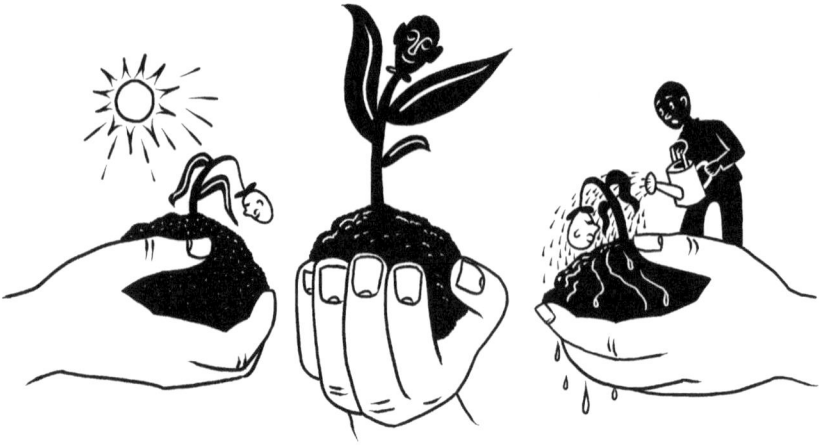

how things end up. This means that while dementia is impacting and affecting a person and those impacts are rippling out to affect those around them, at the same time a whole host of other ripples made by dementia are rippling right back and affecting what dementia is for that person.

This is not in any way unique to dementia. All kinds of systems work this way, increasing our confidence that it's true for dementia too. Work in social-ecological systems, for instance, has noted that the impacts of events in one type of system can have significant implications for other connected types (Xu et al., 2015). Work to improve the resilience of ecological systems, like agricultural systems that farm food crops, is enhanced if the farmers and communities growing that food also have more social and economic resilience. Resilience in systems can lead to further resilience in others (and by extension diminished resilience can likewise be contagious). Intriguingly, this work suggests that perturbations that affect the resilience in one living/social system could improve the sustainability of the complex of systems that are connected to it. If we can increase the resilience in one system or group of systems, we can perhaps support other connected (but dissimilar) systems to achieve the same thing.

This seems to reinforce and clarify Kitwood's important idea that the more we treat people with dementia as if their dementia diminishes or negates them, the more they diminish or are negated (malignant social psychology). At the level of the care network, systems thinking suggests that the resilience (or instability) of that network might impact and lead to further resilience (or instability) within the systems of the person with dementia themselves. Additionally, improving the resilience of the social systems of persons with dementia may also enable them to continue to withstand the challenges that dementia creates over time.

It's worth dwelling on these points a bit more because they're important. Supporting care networks to be more resilient may aid them in remaining care networks even if things get tougher, but, and critically, these resilient care networks may support further resilience in the personal systems of a person with dementia. In other words, improving the resilience of care networks may be a way of changing dementia experiences, a feat which has been achieved by precious few of our tools despite many decades of trying. More fundamentally, however, if, as we've noticed above, we can validly think about dementia as a systems perturbation, something which impacts and disturbs all kinds of systems starting with the mental systems of the person who has the diagnosis, then, being able to support the resilience of social systems around dementia can also be thought of as a direct "treatment" of dementia. By being able to detect systems changes and support resilience in the social networks around a person with dementia, we can potentially improve the dementia experience and do something to improve dementia itself.

PART FOUR
Rethinking dementia

1. Dementia: the rock, the ripple, or the response?

To get to the heart of what systems thinking might mean to dementia, I'd like to begin by posing a question. Throughout this book we've described dementia as involving a neuropathology and series of changes in a person that's like a stone being dropped into a still pool. These changes ripple out, affecting the world around that person in a host of complicated ways. These ripples trigger an even greater and more complex number of responses, resounding echoes of ideas and interpretations about all that has happened which rush back, re-centring, to where the stone fell, crazing the surface of the water in ever more complicated ways. My question then is, "Is dementia the rock, the ripples or the response?"

To keep working this question through, let's return to some ideas we explored a little earlier about what dementia means to people. As we discussed in the first part of this book, people commonly associate dementia with a deterioration and loss of selfhood and of identity, a loss of central, critical parts of how we see ourselves and those we're closest to. We worry about dementia and we're afraid of it happening. For many of us, the dementia experience cannot possibly be tolerable. The costs of what we feel is lost in dementia are simply too high. Adding further weight to our distress, we can't currently know with confidence who dementia will happen to, how to stop it from happening or even reliably delay it. It is no wonder that we are seeing such a focus on "voluntary assisted dying" being available for people with dementia.[41] Arguably, however, our major response to the need to exert power over the dementia experience has been through trying to minimise its effects. This includes the obvious elements of supporting people with a diagnosis to live as well and as safely as possible. More subtly, though, in order to salvage as much as can be saved, it includes a reframing of what dementia has and hasn't done. The primary re-framing mechanism has been through the language of personhood. Encouraging the view that dementia doesn't stop a person being a person helps us to continue to see value in the experience of someone with dementia, and to know what providing care should mean and include. Understandably, we're suggesting that being a person has a value and dignity that should be supported, recognised and protected.[42] We're also suggesting that if personhood continues throughout dementia, then this continuity implies that the person's experiences should still be of value even if, because of the dementia, these experiences seem very different to everyone else's.

Personhood isn't the only idea that people have used to argue that we need to be cautious of dismissing the experiences of people with dementia. The persistence of citizenship and selfhood, for example, are other important aspects of people with dementia that have rightly been identified. In light of the relevance between systems thinking and dementia, however, it is worth taking time to explore how systems thinking changes the relevance of focusing on these ways of understanding and responding to a person with dementia.

As a memory jog (or for anyone who's raced to the back of the book to get the answers) the focus on personhood in dementia was a response to a particular set of problems. The personhood movement was a revolutionary step to subvert "traditional" approaches to understanding dementia as a biomedical illness arising only from medically definable causes (Kitwood, 2019). Kitwood's personhood was edgy in its rebellion against vested (mostly medical) interests and inconsistencies which affected how dementia and those people with the diagnosis were understood and were treated (Dewing, 2008a). By claiming that a persisting and valuable person remained present despite dementia, Kitwood and others were suggesting that we all should be doing more to support that person. They were also making the important claim that how people with dementia were treated had important consequences, including that treating people with dementia as persons (or not) had an impact on their experience and, in effect, what dementia meant for that person (Kitwood, 2019; Sabat & Harré, 1992). While personhood has influenced care for persons with dementia its effect has not always been beneficial. In practice, the person-centred care resulting from a focus on personhood can be more of a homogeneous, tick-box exercise than care that responds to the unique needs of a person (Chapman et al., 2022; Dewing, 2008a). Considering personhood as something that is always present can also have subtly erosive effects on the relevance of that person and on how they are regarded. From this way of understanding personhood, a person doesn't need to do anything to be considered valuable, they always are. This sounds like a good thing unless this status is considered a kind of high-water mark for that person. That is, the person with dementia always remains a person and nothing more. Additionally, because they always have this status, what they think, do, say or experience seems to lose a little relevance. Those people around the person with dementia have decided on their worth and their input into figuring that out is unnecessary. Ironically enough, this focus on personhood can subtly miss hearing from people with dementia about who *they* think they are, and what *they* feel is relevant to them (Chapman et al., 2022).

Personhood isn't the only status that has been afforded and defended for people with dementia. Seeing a person with dementia as a citizen has also been a focus for some thinkers. This focus intends to maintain a special social status for people with dementia to disarm the usual power imbalances which they are often affected by (Bartlett & O'Connor, 2007; Behuniak, 2010; Brijnath & Manderson, 2008). Ideally, this should support and uphold a person with dementia's right to a relevant social self and to act as a valuable participant in the activities of normal society (Phinney et al., 2016).

While being a person or a citizen feels important, it doesn't feel like all that someone with dementia is. From Hilde Lindemann's description of an actor as a way of differentiating some of the roles we inhabit, experience and display for each other, we noted that being a person or a citizen was like a character played by the actor and recognised by the crowd — a status and an identity. The person on stage though isn't just a character, they're an actor. In Lindemann's analogy the actor is our selfhood and the impact of dementia on this facet of ourselves has also been explored. It's been noted that people with dementia have an ongoing experience of themselves, a "mineness" which seems important to them and should be to us. Some have described this as something that relates to their presence and awareness and is connected to their physical body as an "embodied selfhood" which persists even when dementia is advanced (Kontos, 2005). This is an awareness of myself which arises because I remain a physical being, even if dementia has affected many of the mental and communicative aspects of how I may formerly have experienced myself (Sabat, 2002; Sabat & Harré, 1992).

Who are we protecting?

These ideas of identity and personhood are important and helpful ways of exploring what dementia might mean. They focus on the principle that what we need to do is identify and support an aspect of a person with dementia, such as that they remain a valued person or a citizen.

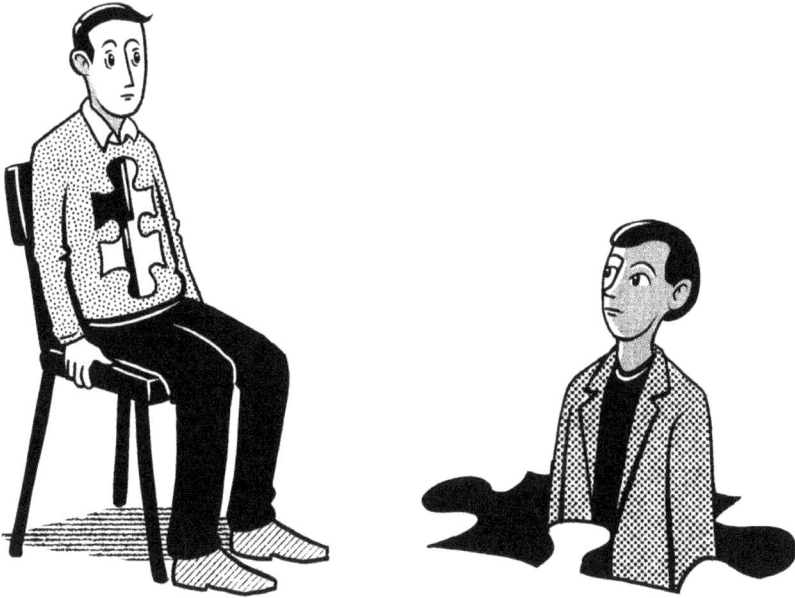

The implication being that, if we can look in the right way, we can find something in the dementia experience which can confidently be said to be unchanged and solid, that the person with dementia is "the same" now as they used to be before dementia was recognised. By doing that, these approaches argue, we can support people with dementia to live as well as they can by taking heart in and nurturing all that there is about them that's not impacted by dementia.

There are clearly some important truths here. It seems natural and reassuring to look for and expect the familiar in others, regardless of dementia. But should that really be our focus? This question is interesting and important to me. I think "personhood" suggests a solidification and continuity within dementia which is clearly attractive and reassuring. However, if we understand those qualities as antidotes to dementia's problems, what we also seem to be saying is that dementia is by contrast a state of fracturing and discontinuity. While a focus on personhood is thought of as an approach which maintains and supports key aspects of a person with dementia, I wonder whether it might also represent a missed opportunity for us to engage with how things change in dementia in more positive ways.

A more fertile, if challenging, approach to thinking about dementia is through systems thinking. From a systems perspective, someone with dementia is not (and was never) a whole, continuous and unchanging person. They were, and are, a complex of interacting systems. Dementia starts pathologies with various processes changing the workings of circuits within our brains. We fear dementia, at least in part, because so much of how we see ourselves and others, and so much that we associate as being valuable about us seems tied up with how we think. But people don't reside in their brains. Disturbing the neurological make up of a person can be a big change, but our brain is just part of who we are, not all of it.

We are made up multiple types of interacting systems. Fascinatingly, we don't experience ourselves like this. An amazing quirk of our experience is that the result of all these systems interacting with each other is our familiar (and, ironically, shared) experience of being a singular, independent, rational, autonomous individual. A large contributor to this for many of us in a particular culture is the emphasis on this individual experience being normal, good and valued. Tragically, the devotion towards this view of our world probably compounds our distress and maximises everything that is disrupted when these tenuous fantasies are filtered away by dementia.[43]

We started this section focusing again on notions of "self", "identity" or "personhood." The point was not to suggest that these aren't important or valuable ideas or states, but rather to try and get to what lies underneath these words and see what that can teach us. Systems thinking would suggest that self, identity and personhood are experiences which emerge from the "world-making" interaction of our physical, conscious/mental, communicative and social systems.[44] Our conscious/mental systems develop and increase in complexity as we grow and learn. These mental systems are also "structurally coupled" (connected and mutually reactive) with communicative systems of interaction, and thereby with a larger world of social systems and systems of ideas which provide frameworks and language for our experiences. "Identity", "selfhood" and "personhood" are experiences arising from these coupled systems. They are experiences that I recognise and that are recognised by others. They are experiences which develop and shift in shared meanings during the course of a life, emerging as ideas and interpretations from systems of words and language. My identity is not a singular or static mental thing that I possess, but a lifelong development among the people with an experience of me, and closely tied to the language we use to share and describe these ideas. My mental world itself, while clearly mine and therefore associated with me as an individual, is also completely inseparable from these other interconnected systemic experiences. We all will and do continuously influence each other.

Dementia is another factor, disruptive and destructive as it might be, within this mix of interconnection and responsiveness. It's no wonder then that dementia's impact is complex and enigmatic. It clearly does affect mental, communicative and social systems in significant ways. But it also doesn't affect us in the way we often think it does. Collectively, we aren't victims of the unstoppable monster of dementia. We (as the result of connected systems) participate very actively in deciding what dementia is and means. Identity can assuredly be affected by dementia, but a continuous or reliable identity was never available to us in the first place, and therefore won't be lost due to dementia's impact. Dementia changes people's already changing identities, rather than introducing a dynamic into something static and predictable. These new avenues of change in dementia also don't have to mean disconnection in a fundamental sense. This is because systems undergo constant change and are always coupled to their environments and other systems. Dementia's impact on the systems relating to a person or people doesn't mean that these systems are no longer interacting with each other. In fact, our uncertainties in trying to understand what "identity", "selfhood" or "personhood" mean in dementia or in testing how well terms like "citizen", "monster", "partner" or "parent" fit a person with dementia reveal just how interconnected these systems are and how deep an impact dementia can have on all of us.

Knowing that systems change as a natural part of how they work can be comforting — if only that this awareness makes the idea that experiences that arise from systems like being a "self" or a "person" also change seem more commonplace and less confronting. Systems change constantly but in doing so they usually also remain recognisable. Living systems have a "circular organisation", meaning that they remain the same system despite change, usually because they continue having the same function(s), despite changes in structure. The presence of dementia will lead to (additional) perturbations within systems but does not automatically mean that a system will be completely different.

As we explored in "Systems and complexity", change within systems can potentially result in resilience or disruption depending on the context of the systems in question. Each person is the result, not of a single system but of multiple systems. Some of these systems are personal and connected to us, like the systems of our physical bodies, and others are more dispersed, like those including how communities and societies engage with a person. Changes in one system can perturb others, but this does not automatically result in the system losing its circular organisation. As an example, if a community feels that the experience of a person with dementia is meaningless, that might affect how members of that community act towards the person with dementia. This might have a negative impact on the experiences of that person with dementia; however, it won't dictate that a person with dementia's experiences have no meaning for them. Rich and complex experiences and meaning may persist within the systems changes of dementia, despite the behaviour of others.

This relates to a further observation that living systems determine their own responses to the experiences that perturb them. They have structural plasticity. They are able to learn and respond to their environment (H. Maturana & Varela, 1980). Due to these qualities, living systems are autonomous and self-determined (Dell, 1985). People with dementia remain autonomous in their plastic responsiveness to their experiences, even when their diagnosis is advanced. Nellie reflected on the "art" of showing care through physically providing for her children; Patrick created still life variations for an audience of one; and April relived her connection to the songs and dances of her youth and her family. People with advanced dementia engage with and explore their worlds, it's just that their efforts are often discounted in comparison with what would be expected from a normal "person", like the one we believe they used to be. Mandy, Patrick and April were all still recognisable through the way they continued to respond and adapt to their worlds. They were still recognisable as living human people. They weren't the same. Dementia had clearly had an impact on the normal changes in systems that had led to those moments, but the systems and the people were still recognisable.

And this point, perhaps, takes us to the crux of what I think we needed to think through together. If people with dementia are always changing (as all people do), and if those people continue to be present in their changing fashion during dementia, what is it about dementia that is so terrifying? What is it that seems different and challenging from this experience? Why are we so troubled by the particular changed systems and changed selves that the dementia experience involves?

We've explored many potential answers to that question, such as how prone we are to fearing dependence and our worry that dementia represents a fundamental type of descent and loss of control. But, again, I think there might be another level to this towards which systems thinking seems to guide. Living systems work due to their independent but responsive connection to other systems and their environment, their structural coupling. Unless a system remains structurally coupled to its environment it will eventually dissolve and dissipate. There are no solitary living systems. We/they all rely on relationships and interconnection to continue to function and to be. Perhaps the experiences of people with dementia are such a source of worry and uncertainty for everyone because we recognise that their coupling to all that is around them has changed. They remain connected to us; we can be sure of that. Their living, breathing, responsive, communicative, affecting persistence means that they remain connected to their world, and to the systems that create it. The experience of people with dementia moves and motivates us. The evidence is all around us. The fact that I took the time to write this book and you the time to read it, in addition to innumerable other moments and accounts trying to get to the bottom of what dementia means, shows us how very connected to dementia we are. But dementia changes the nature and the manner of connection. Perhaps the primary impact of dementia, through its complicated, rippling impact, is to affect how people with dementia connect to themselves, to those around them, to systems of meaning and language — how they "fit" into their world.

Old systems, new fit

Fitting into our world is a complex business. Using the metaphor of us fitting like puzzle pieces, slotting and sliding into and around each other seems tempting, but a dance is probably a better image. We all constantly shift and step to shape and maintain our place within the maelstrom of movement of our colossal, encompassing partner — every other living system. In this vast waltz, every living system moves and responds to all the others. Dementia is here in this dance with us. Dementia is something that is experienced, but it is also something that is responded to. It's something that impacts how the dancers move with each other, the form and fit of our human systems.

We describe dementia as a disease, a feared descent, a change to cognition and communication, a reason to consider suicide, an enemy to be vanquished, a prison, a threat to societies' resource management, a political opportunity, a philosophical dilemma, and a myriad of other ideas. Rather than being one thing, dementia includes all these descriptions and understandings, it's a web of meanings and ideas constituted from many sources. When a person is "diagnosed" with dementia it's a name being given to a variety of changes and influences in their social and personal systems, the catalyst usually being microscopic changes within that person's brain. But this diagnosed dementia isn't something that is just described or categorised, it is something that is directly experienced by those people closest to it. There's an important potential separation here between dementia as an experience and dementia as an idea. Both clearly have an effect on each other within the web of systems impacts we've been exploring, but they also don't seem to be exactly the same thing. We began this book reflecting on the many reasons dementia is described in the ways that it is, prior to focusing more specifically on how it's experienced. What can we learn now about our descriptions of dementia given our recognition that systems are central to dementia's impact?

A starting point is to note that this system of ideas and descriptions of dementia are just that, another system which responds and changes. The chief focus of this system of ideas is to make sense of the impact and the experience of dementia; and a lot of other different systems and ideas have an influence on this. Evidence for this is how much our understanding of dementia has changed and continues to change. Even the definition of dementia is changing. What we consider as the diagnostic criteria for dementia — what's needed to be present for us to agree that the word "dementia" applies or doesn't — has changed a lot over time. Neurobiologically, we're still putting the pieces together, trying to figure out what ideas fit into the dementia jigsaw, and which don't. Many of the most obvious changes that have occurred have been driven by research and technology. The experience of dementia is being understood using lenses previously unavailable to us. There's been incremental shifts in understanding what dementia means and involves, a lot of which may not have led to a great change in the broad sweep of this system of ideas. While it will be important to clarify the neuropathological specifics underlying dementia, it's likely that these details may not be that meaningful for many people. Regarding the scientific and medical ideas that we use to understand dementia, more influential is probably the limited change in options for treatment that clarifications in neuropathology have resulted in for the vast majority of people. We're also more confident that scientific changes mean that we can better predict who might get dementia, while nevertheless still feeling that dementia is what you have or you don't have based on the expert clinical judgement of someone who may or may not utilise newer medical tests.

A dementia diagnosis is considered as something different from "normal" or from other versions of a risky "near-normal" such as "pre-dementia" or "mild cognitive impairment", even while the arbitrary lines that determine these categories have continued to change. Despite constant change and progress influencing the development of this system of ideas relating to dementia, the result is a stabilising diagnostic sense of dementia, an increasing confidence in what dementia means from a medical and scientific point of view even while new meanings of the spaces around dementia have started to be created with dementia beginning to be understood as existing alongside some sort of non-dementia state. The implications of these developments have likely been tempered by the continuous shared concern that, regardless of whether these states are called dementia or mild-cognitive impairment, there's only a limited amount we can currently do medically to change them.

Dementia means more to us than just a diagnosis or a definition. Actually, it's probably more correct to say that dementia *is* more than just a diagnosis or a definition; and thinking that dementia is a kind of yes or no binary is problematic. Our understanding of our experience is shaped by culture and language, and objective truths are rare (Haraway, 2015; Irigaray, 1985). This is not to challenge the relevance of the clinical diagnosis of dementia, but to point out that the label may include more than we intend, and that it may not always mean the same thing. This system of meanings of dementia includes everything that contributes to how we understand the dementia experience, and what it means to have dementia or care for someone with it. This system of meanings is influenced by very subtle things, tiny ripples that bounce and build, resulting in something different. These ideas are not static and fixed but are constantly shifting and changing. The meanings that arise from one way of understanding and engaging with dementia influence the whole of what we're left with. When we talk about dementia in different ways, for example, when dementia is discussed economically as a colossal and worrying drain on resources, or legally as a vulnerability needing authorisation of others to make decisions, or politically as a cause for advocacy to wage in a heroic battle, or societally as an inescapable loss that's deeply feared, we're witnessing both the result of dementia's changing meaning and the process that supports bringing that about. Within the various and complex systems of meaning which make up our world, a diagnosis of dementia is not "information," but interpretation.[45] "Dementia" validly means all of our popular (and troubling) views on the topic, including that people with dementia don't have autonomy, are victims, zombies, or any other variation. The label of "dementia" means a vast number of potential things (including our changeable neurobiological understanding), it is subject to the interpretation of the human systems that make these judgements, and dementia, ultimately, means to those systems what they, the systems, think it does.

Within the constant dance, the ripple and response of systems, the system of meanings of dementia is changing continuously. It's not alone in this. Changing systems of meaning are everywhere. One that I think about a lot that's related to the dementia experience is our ideas and expectations about death and dying. The increased global focus on deaths that happen when people choose to die using medical intervention to bring death about (called voluntary assisted dying [VAD] in Australia and a variety of other terms elsewhere) could be seen as signifying a shift or transformation in the systems of meaning related to ideas of what we think "normal" or "good" dying means (Collier 2023). I'm not suggesting that it's bad or wrong to have access to VAD or to use VAD, but rather that the very possibility of VAD in the way that it exists now reflects changes in what we think "good" dying means to us. The relationship of VAD and "good" dying to dementia is that there is a growing interest in many places in exploring some means to extend VAD legislation to allow people with dementia to have access to these choices. You may be reading this surprised that people with dementia can't already easily access VAD. The reasons they aren't are complicated and beyond the scope of this book. We can, however, focus them down to the challenge of applying the notion of a voluntary decision for dying in advanced illness to people with dementia who, due to the impacts of dementia, may be unable to express clearly a voluntary request for VAD, or an experience of suffering, when their dementia is advanced and their decision-making capacity is impaired. The reason for raising VAD as an issue isn't to dig into the pros or cons of people with dementia having access to VAD, but to highlight that the fact that there's a lot of interest in VAD being available in dementia suggests something about what it means to get sick and die with dementia. One possible systems-framed interpretation of this phenomenon is that systems of meaning of dementia, including the fairly stable worries that dementia is to be feared — that it represents an inhuman and undignified experience and that there's nothing that can be done to fix it — has had a significant impact on this other system of ideas grappling with what "good" dying means. This has played a role in an emerging transformation whereby the only way that dying with dementia might result in a "good" death is if VAD is involved.

These sorts of general observations about how big collective and responsive systems of meanings work — and the directions they're moving in — is, unfortunately, of limited relevance. There may be some truth to what I've said about what dementia means at the time of writing but, equally, a lot will have changed by the time you read this. The ripples would have continued to spread and shift. Not everything will have changed. As we've learned together, systems often stay the same despite constantly changing because they continue to have the same function. I'm confident that we'll still have a system of ideas for what we think dementia means even allowing for the time that it has taken me to have this book published. There will also likely be some consistency in the functions of this system of dementia meanings. The system might have many functions, but I think a central one is probably to try to understand the challenge of dementia, to figure out and place dementia somewhere so we can all know how worried we need to be about it. Assuming that this is true, means something about everything that has been discussed in this book. What we hear, see and read about dementia, about how it works neuro-biologically, about the experiences of people who have it or who care for people with dementia, about the routinely poor treatment that people with dementia receive in aged care currently, is not us receiving information.[46] All of these ideas and experiences are influences, perturbations, which are incorporated into our individual and collective sense of what dementia means. Sometimes these pile up to radically transform what dementia means to us all. The initial neuro-biological diagnosis of dementia and the corresponding sense that it was a singular and therefore fixable problem was clearly a transformative force in what dementia meant. The more recent and decided loss of an optimistic meaning of dementia has remained stable despite a myriad of important small changes. Dementia's current meaning seems to be characterised by fear, isolation, de-valuing, and disregard. We could even dispiritingly observe that this seems to be becoming increasingly true. The example discussed above about how dying with dementia is regarded seems to be evidence of this. Despite the lifelong efforts of many thinkers, writers, carers, policy makers, scientists, advocates and others, our systems of the meaning of dementia have seemed resilient to the many influences that they've thrown into the mix to try to improve how and what we value in dementia. All this effort seems to have resulted in a common and reinforcing (first order) response to our troubled ideas about the meaning of dementia. If you'll permit the expression, I think our cumulative systemic response to these problems has been "de-moralised". It's a response that knows that things aren't getting better but reasonably and defensively notes that we are doing the best we can.

It's easy to feel disappointed. But it's also important to remember that this isn't the whole story. New interpretations, new challenges, the right influence at the right time, can lead to transformation (Lyotard, 1979). Kitwood's nurturing the personhood of people with dementia, Kontos's highlighting the importance of the selves of people with dementia within their physical body and responses, the United Nations Convention on the Rights of People with Disabilities, the Royal Commission into Aged Care in Australia and many other landmarks and ideas have led to important changes and transformations (some major, and some minor) resulting in new ways of understanding dementia in some spheres and areas. The limited degree of transformation in our systems of the meaning of dementia since these interventions does not indicate a "failure" of these ideas or landmarks but should remind us that systems determine their own responses. These ideas and challenges fit how we understood dementia at that time to influence it in the way that they did. Specific changes cannot be forced on systems. Systems don't work like that. The somewhat disheartening lack of transformation in how we understand dementia does not mean that change is impossible, just that it hasn't happened yet.

Steps towards an ecology of dementia

Returning to our question about whether dementia is the rock, the ripples or the responses, you've probably guessed that I think dementia includes all of these things and all the changeable and responsive ways that they can influence each other. This seems a long way from what Alzheimer and others proposed when they were framing our more contemporary ideas about dementia. However, it may be that rethinking dementia in this way, as something arising from different systems influencing each other, provides resources for responding to dementia differently and improving things further.

As we've discussed, what is thought of as "dementia" is a complex interaction between multiple systems. While on the one hand we can say that the experience of dementia is a different thing from how that dementia is described and understood, on the other hand, they're inseparably interlinked. The experience of dementia starts with a whole cascade of changes and influences in a person's mental, physical and communicative systems. Subtle changes in memory, language or personality might be what we feel or notice but these experiences themselves are just the bits that we can appreciate from all kinds of systems working within us and around us all the time, largely without our notice. These changes only really become dementia, and are called by this term, when they're interpreted through a variety of other different ways of making sense of these experiences — systems in themselves that are the social and clinical ways of describing and categorising what's happening. What the dementia diagnosis is felt to mean is also influenced by all sorts of other dynamic systems of culture, language, economics, politics, what we consider knowledge, what we consider the meaning of experience and what we consider as caring. Dementia cannot solely be "a clinical syndrome", as the diagnostic criteria for dementia provide just the barest hint of everything that the word implies and relates to. Dementia exists as something created and experienced through the interwoven effects of perturbed living systems and their environments. Dementia is best understood as an eco-system.

This is, I know, a strange position to take for someone who is a medical doctor and in the practice of diagnosing and treating diseases. But taking an ecological view of dementia leads to some surprising and useful ideas. Gregory Bateson was a writer and thinker who trained as an anthropologist but contributed to many different fields. He described the concept of mind in ecological terms (Bateson, 1972a; Oliveira, 2013). Mind isn't a single thing, it is a result of interactions, and arises from ideas and language systems through which we understand and describe our world (Bateson, 1972a). In this sense, we can't separate mind from the process used to think about what it is and describe it. It is not a discrete organ but a dynamic context that develops even as it is perceived. Mind is not static. It is a process that always travels to an unreached horizon, an *ad-mentia* (or towards-mind). It is a constant exploration and interpretation, ever changing and effecting change.

A significant proportion of what is encompassed by Bateson's notion of mind would be changed by dementia. Ideas, language and experiences, the substrates of mind, are influenced and potentially diminished or obscured by dementia, but the interactive, energetic and responsive quality of mind continues. This is a difficult idea to feel comfortable with in the face of all the change that dementia involves. Even the name "dementia" leads us off track. "Dementia", however, is not a *de-mentia* (away from mind); it is not a separation, a descent or a negation of mind. Dementia perturbs what's involved in mind, changing its form and how it is perceived, but it does not extinguish it. It does not stop its movement, its *ad-mentia*. As mind arises ecologically through connections between the exploring, thinking processes of a being and their world it is and remains more than the discrete and affected mental process of the person with dementia. The experience of dementia and of mind arises from the responsive, communicative connections between personal mental systems and the surrounding world. The root biological causes that give rise to dementia change the "fit" and flow of these connections, but they do not remove them. Gautama Siddhartha (the Buddha) said "mind is everything". Mind is everywhere and is everything that we are. Dementia as a perturbation, an influenced mental ecology is similarly inescapable. From everywhere that we try and think of dementia, it's there already, the ideas, questions and uncertainties influencing how we might think about and respond to this kind of challenge. We can't be outside the influence that dementia has and does have on all of us.

This ecological view of dementia brings existing ideas into new focus. Kitwood controversially suggested that "*re-mentia*" (a return to mind) might be possible for those with the diagnosis (Dewing, 2008a). Kitwood was proposing the idea that the right conditions might mean that the changes of dementia could be turned back, leading to an increased capacity of communication, feeling or learning. An ecological view of dementia would suggest that this might not be possible and, more controversially, might not be necessary. I'm not saying that what we observe as the "pathological" changes of dementia in tests, investigations and behaviour of dementia will always be the same, or that we will never be able to come up with a treatment or influence that will change them. Far from it. I'm certain that we will. But despite this, dementia will have had an impact on us. Systems change and develop but they don't return to where they were. If I stop watering a sapling tree and then begin again, it may recover, the living system adapting to the period of want and then subsequent plenty. But the adaptations will remain etched in its fabric, in the eventual rings of its physical history. Changes have occurred and "improvement" does not erase the system's historical development. Additionally, Kitwood's hope for a *re-mentia* implies the recovery of something lost, but the ecological mind is not lost in dementia. It is changed. What Kitwood implies here is a return to what was past but, as we've discussed, the movement of mind (and of systems) is ceaseless and, while systems may become more stable and function more securely, they don't return to their own past.

A world of words

It is primarily through language that responses to the ripples of dementia and explorations of what dementia means take place. How we talk about dementia reflects what we think and feel about it. But the language we use in response to dementia is also part of the systems that form what dementia means to us, and like all systems this language can change. Change may actually be something we should seek or at least explore when it comes to language. Challenging our assumptions through actively thinking through the language we use to describe things can help us shift and deepen our understanding of what we're saying and what we're meaning (Bateson, 1972a). We talked earlier in this book about the language used for dementia as being a barometer for how we feel about it. Bateson, however, posits language not just as a barometer but as a thermostat. Within an ecological view of dementia, thinking through language can be a step toward modifying it, and modifying language can be a step towards influencing the dementia experience.

As we've noted, we commonly use linguistic devices, like metaphor, when we talk and think about dementia. The use of these sorts of devices reveals a lot about the ecological workings of dementia, about what dementia means to us, and what's at stake. The scale and the threat within the language we use to convey dementia is noteworthy. Catastrophic metaphors are common. In writing, dementia is often an unstoppable natural force (like a flood or tidal wave) that we, as individuals and as a society, are powerless to resist. Dementia is also an unimaginable un-death, with zombies who have an eerie resemblance to those we love but are ultimately a threat to be feared (Behuniak, 2011). Due to the penetration of these associations, dementia is now a metonym for doom; dementia means catastrophe (Zeilig, 2014). Our fear of dementia has not stopped us making use of it. Language is used to influence how we think about dementia and how we behave in response to it. The disaster of dementia has been explored in popular media, entertainment and in policy approaches to the problem. Burke has suggested that this exploration can reflect a politics that seeks to draw power from vulnerability (Burke, 2016). In this way, the use of language to describe dementia allows a position of moral and political power. Alternate perspectives are side-lined through a bullish "with us or against us" approach that does not engage with these complexities. Interestingly, these ideas are not unique to the ecology of dementia. George and Whitehouse describe the metaphoric similarities between the "War on terror" and the "War on Alzheimer's Disease" (George & Whitehouse, 2014). In both these cases, fear of catastrophe requires aggressive (and costly) responses to an enemy from which society needs protection. This frequent use of catastrophic language seems linked to the pursuit of social, political, and economic purposes within the ecology of dementia. It's worth wondering what a different approach to how we describe dementia might mean and what the results might be.

It's also notable that these sorts of language choices have implications beyond just what dementia means. As an ecosystem of meanings, the language we choose and use for dementia (a state that we consider as being a pathology, or something that isn't "normal") may influence or reflect how we think and talk about our many "normal" frailties and dependencies. The language we use for dementia can act as a "lens through which we might be able to see" what we think about ourselves and our lives more clearly — raising the possibility that understanding and responding to dementia may have a deeper and more fundamental meaning than you might expect (Zeilig, 2014).

A lot of what is said about dementia represents and expresses a fear of being overwhelmed, forgotten and left behind. In language and literature dementia represents the struggle we feel to keep up to date with what's important personally and collectively. In Tony Harrison's poem, *The Mother of the Muses*, or even more obliquely, in Kazuo Ishiguro's 2015 novel, *The Buried Giant*, dementia is the foil that enables an exploration of our societies' tendency to forget and move on from, rather than to overcome, its challenges. Trevor Smith's play, *An Evening with Dementia*, demonstrates that the disconnected, vulnerable and victimised experience of dementia shares a commonality with "normal" experiences in society. Within this ecology of experiences, "A person with dementia is only separate from the rest of us by virtue of a medical diagnosis" (Zeilig, 2014). Dementia seems to reside in a paradoxical space as something that gets under our skin, not because it's alien and inexplicable but because it is worryingly familiar, an echo of how we live and how we age. This seems the case in Jonathan Franzen's, *The Corrections*, where dementia seems to act as part of the myriad of forces creating our complex and interconnected world. Perhaps our ideas about dementia demonstrate the frailty, fragility and powerlessness which we often feel but wish to reject and side-line as abnormality.

There may be an extra step that we could take here relating to language choices and what they mean. This idea, that aspects of our language relating to dementia might express our fears about our normal experiences, makes even the idea of dementia being a "pathology" seem worthy of exploring. There is another way of engaging with this baseline way of categorising dementia. We could wonder whether what we see and experience in dementia is only understandable as a pathology or whether it could be better described as an adaptation. Explaining this seemingly controversial idea requires us to think a little about the lenses we use to understand the systemic experience of a health problem. When I have a cold a lot of what I experience as illness is actually my body's response to the viral infection. The two are interlinked phenomena where what I experience and describe as illness is simultaneously my various body systems' attempts at healing, normalising and repair. This idea doesn't mean that there isn't a problem (the virus) contributing to what's happening, but at the same time a lot of what we experience as having a cold is actually systemic responses to this problem and not the problem itself. Could the same be true with dementia? Mitchell and Snyder explore this way of viewing "pathology" through a highly personal and scholarly article they wrote responding to their family's experience. Mitchell and Snyder's daughter (Emma) was born with a significant disability, a diagnosis called oesophageal atresia where a person is born without part of the oesophagus (Mitchell & Snyder, 2016). In their article, Mitchell and Snyder call for Emma's disability and those like it not to be seen just as a failure of her body to build itself in a normal way. They suggest instead that her experiences are more correctly her body's attempts to adapt to the negative impact of environmental influences like water pollution and medical mismanagement. The fact that this adaptive response wasn't able to normalise the challenges Emma's body was faced with doesn't, from their perspective, diminish what was being attempted. Dementia, most usually a neuro-cognitive condition associated with increasing age is clearly different from a disability present at birth. However, the core observation that a lot of what we tend to call "pathology" can also be seen as a body, mind or person's systemic responses to environmental challenges, seems a valid echo of much that has been discussed in this book. It's worth noting here that "environmental" doesn't refer to the physical or natural landscape necessarily, but the things outside the system that we're interested in, that the system is being influenced by. This hints at a fairly radical way of rethinking dementia. How different would dementia seem if we could see some of what's occurring in this light — if the dementia experience was understood to consist of a person and their community's adaptive (rather than pathological) responses to change? If dementia was a syndrome involving a constellation of social, mental, and psychological attempts to adapt to changing environments. One of the environments creating change would clearly be the microscopic neuro-biological changes that we're so keen to reverse. But another would also probably include all of the social, cultural, and language-based challenges that we've been discussing together. Maybe a new way of thinking about dementia is to try and relax our grip on this notion of it being a terrible pathology and make some space for it actually also being a fragile and imperfect attempt at healing in the most difficult of circumstances.

Healing dementia

Perhaps this is an idea that could help us reconfigure what we think about dementia. As an adaptation, dementia doesn't happen to a person, dementia is an experience that arises from a person and their community as a response to change. It's triggered by neurobiological changes, but the diagnosis and the experience of dementia itself actually manifest from all of the impact on, and the responses of, the systems which engage with those changes (like a person's mental and psychological systems) and from the responsive interconnections between these personal systems and a broader ecology of other systems like the social systems of that person and systems of culture and language that underlie all of this while it's happening. It's the systems affected by dementia that define and create the experience, not the pathological taxonomy that clinicians and scientists work on and use. Dementia is our collaborative, collective response to these changes when they occur for people. In other words, "dementia" is what happens when these neuro-biological triggers occur within the sorts of systems that most of us have available to us, and when those systems are doing their best to respond to these changes.

While challenging, these ideas also hold the seeds of alternative and, I think, empowering ways of rethinking dementia. The ecological consensus that dementia represents pathology is closely related to how cognitive, memory and language changes are associated with diminished worth (Behuniak, 2011). We all know this, and no one wants to be worthless. Consequently, memory loss has become a trigger for fear in every ageing person (Post, 2006). But dementia as an adaptation (rather than a pathology) could be seen as part of the unfolding development of our own situated and complex life-journey rather than as a devastating pathology that is to be fixed and feared. From this perspective, dementia would no longer be diagnosed but revealed and explored by the person themselves, along with the contribution of their community around them. An ecological view of dementia would recognise that it is the person with the diagnosis who is the primary person who is responding to dementia, not the doctor or the aged-care system. The unique human experience of dementia is the first level of adaptation, of attempted healing and making sense of dementia. But it doesn't stop there. This person's experience is the foundational ecological perturbation that influences and stirs everything and everyone around them and is also the most important contributor to ongoing change. As part of the everything and everyone else around them, though, we all have a potential contribution to seeing dementia as adaptation rather than pathology. Our usual, current collective responses to dementia can transform with the right kind of influence. Worrying about the additive potential harms that a "war on dementia" as a "monstrous" descent may cause could be the start towards us approaching this differently. Viewing dementia as an adaption to change (an attempt at healing) may counter-intuitively make this more and more true if it helps us set aside some of the potentially harmful and traumatic interpretations and responses that we commonly assume to be the only ones we have available to us.

If we're talking about dementia as something that's consistent with the idea of adapting and healing, then it seems important to talk a little more about our wish to "cure" dementia. Within the ecology of dementia, the determined quest for a "cure" rather than additional focus on healing dementia, makes no sense. Our approach to living and our successful ageing puts us more at risk of the diagnosis of dementia (George & Whitehouse, 2014; Richards & Brayne, 2010). From this way of looking at things, dementia is an outcome of the accumulated effect of particular ways of living in our world. Like the neurobiological changes that lead to dementia, the fix for dementia would be a system perturbation and nothing more. Multiple attempts to cure or negate specific problems related to dementia have made this clear. We try to fix problems that we see dementia causing when we place dependent people in care facilities, or when we provide those without capacity with surrogate decision-makers. These acts perturb and influence the ecology of dementia, but they don't stop dementia or take away its impact. If (hopefully in the very near future) the neuro-biological changes of dementia could be halted or even reversed, with a pill or therapy, those affected by it would still be changed by the experience. The adaptive response of the dementia experience has and is creating a new existence which has different experiences and meanings as a result of what has occurred. We cannot be "re-constructed" through intervention (Mitchell & Snyder, 2016). Even if we could determine a genetic key for dementia or some other intervention meaning that we would, as a society, never have to diagnose someone with dementia again, dementia would have changed us. Further change does not rewind our responses to our environment and recreate how we were prior to what's happened (as individuals or as a society). Further change makes us anew. So, working for some sort of treatment that meaningfully changes the neuro-biological changes underlying dementia is, of course, an amazing and important aim and one that I and many other people hope will be successful as soon as possible. But we shouldn't think that this will fix all the challenges that dementia raises for us. After such a eureka moment we may find that we've swapped one set of challenges and problems for others. Worse still, we might, if we've been blinkered in our focus on that goal, have missed an opportunity and a need to grow and heal in ways that are really important.

Someday in the future these words will be out of date, and we will have found the interventions we need to fix (at least some of) what we consider dementia. But that won't be a return to some sort of elusive normality. A cure is attractive, in part because its pursuit supports the continued societal focus on the value of individual autonomy. By focusing on curing dementia, we can keep telling ourselves and each other that we are all autonomous in the way that we value, but that's never really been true. We are all interconnected, fragile and dynamic. Individual autonomy, in the way we've been taught by society to value it, was a dream, and one with a growing legacy of problems that it's responsible for. Interestingly, though, a biological cure would not remove the challenges to these values that dementia makes apparent. While I hope that a cure is just around the corner, there's also the possibility that such an intervention will help and hurt us simultaneously. Currently, the magnitude of the challenge of dementia means that we can't help but take notice. The enormity of the task makes me hopeful that learning and growth is likely for us as people and communities. If a rapid medical solution (or the appearance of one) arrived, it may be that the need to think, grow and change would be less. My hope would be for a Goldilocks balance of the best medical solutions as soon as we can and dramatic work as a society not knowing that such a solution is just around the corner. But even after the solution has arrived and the Nobel prizes awarded, dementia will remain with us. Dementia has changed us as a global people, and its impact will continue to be with us, regardless.

Stepping forward

Thinking about healing dementia systems also seems to open some new doors and reveals new possibilities for how we could help promote and sustain adapting in response to dementia's challenges. If dementia is the changes and responses of systems to certain types of neuro-biological changes within an ecology, this means that all manner of things might be able to influence these systems and improve the stability of what's occurring. The complexity of this understanding of dementia may mean it's difficult to know where to start in order to have an impact. The upside here is that the reach and interconnection of the systems involved in what dementia means to us all means that there are very few invalid areas to explore.

If you've got to this point in the book, hopefully you'll allow me to make some sweeping suggestions about ideas that might be helpful in engaging with and improving dementia care systems. In commenting on these, though, I'd remind you again that *systems* determine what they're influenced by. It may be that none or only some of the ideas below are meaningful to the systems you're engaged with and I'm not in any way trying to assume your experience or suggest easy answers.

For *people with dementia*, please know that I am not trying to pretend that I know what you are going through. I and the others around you can't but we'll do everything we can to listen and to help. Sometimes you might feel as though you're on the journey alone. You're not. We're all here with you, we just don't understand what you're feeling and experiencing the way that you do. Knowing that you're not alone might feel reassuring and worrying at the same time. You might be hoping that you'll protect your family from some of what you think is coming. That's an understandable and incredibly noble and loving way to be feeling, but it was never going to be that way. Dementia has always been around and affects us all even when we're not aware of it. Its impact for you and your family is clearer now because of your diagnosis but we could never completely escape how it has touched the communities we live in. That's the nature of this kind of experience. So, if we can't protect each other from these things, then the next best thing might be to do our best to share and be open with each other, to try and support each other in whatever way we're able. The great thing about that kind of sharing is that it's never too late to start or to do more. Whatever feels right for you will be the right way to do it.

For *people with dementia*, please be assured that we all know that this isn't your fault. We know that you didn't choose this and we're all doing our best to adapt and learn even while everything keeps changing. We know that you are working and trying as hard as you're able. If you have ideas about what might help, why not share them with someone around you? Maybe even the sharing will feel different and positive. If there are things that you're hoping for or things that you're worried about, why don't we talk about those too. Maybe knowing more about what you're hoping for will allow others to feel confident that they are indeed helping in the way they want to. And, maybe planning for a few of the things you're worried about will mean that you can put those worries down and not have to carry them with you all the time. Are there other things that you could think about like that? You might feel like a lot has changed or even that you've lost much of what you felt was key to who you are over time due to the dementia. Sometimes thinking and worrying about the things we feel we've lost can end up becoming another heavy load to carry. Maybe you don't have to do that alone, or maybe that's another load we can set aside if we talk about it. Maybe that might help lessen the worry. Everyone's way of doing that is different, but talking to others about how you feel about what's changed might be a start.

For *people with dementia*, maybe you've found your carer(s) or your healthcare providers pretty frustrating to deal with. You wouldn't be alone. Know that they're also trying really hard and using the best ideas they've got to try to help. Just like you, they don't have a map. Maybe you can help each other figure out the next steps? If you've got ideas about how you would like to be involved in any decisions that might need to be made, perhaps it would be good to talk about that too. Not because anyone knows that there's anything big or urgent on the horizon, but because sometimes we're so used to being alongside the main people in our lives that we forget to check in with how we work together and how we support each other when things are changing. Most of all, know that you are loved and treasured now, just as you've always been. If there's more that we can do to remind you of that just let us know.

For *carers*, please know that you are doing an absolutely spectacular job. Most of us don't volunteer to be carers, it just happens because we're people who care about someone, about others, and then they need us more. If you're ever not sure what to do, what to say, or that you aren't sure you've got enough to keep giving, know that you aren't on your own. Finding the energy to ask or reach out for help is a huge challenge, I know, but I also know that it can get easier from there if we take that first step. Maybe give it a try.

For *carers*, I've learned from my work that dementia means that someone changes. It doesn't mean we lose the person they used to be, but it also doesn't mean that they stay the same. They have that history of being that person from before and the one they are now. You've probably changed in lots of ways too, I'm sure, but seeing the sometimes dramatic changes in someone we care about can be really difficult. Realising that your relationship with the person you care for is different, or that you're dealing with them differently now doesn't mean that you're doing it wrong. That's a natural response to all those changes. Maybe you've found the person you care for or your healthcare providers pretty frustrating to deal with. You wouldn't be alone. Know that they're trying and using the best ideas and tools they've got. Just like you, they don't have a map. Maybe you can help each other figure out the next step? If it feels safe to do so, you could have a conversation about what's changed with the person you care for and see where that leads. If that's not a good idea but you have something to say, finding someone else to talk to — a friend or family member, another carer, someone from your own health team — might be a good idea instead. Remember you won't be able to keep caring for them unless you're also caring for you. If things aren't working with the person you're caring for it's worth wondering "is there something that I can do differently that might help?" Sometimes a small change can have a big impact. If not, remember that what's needed may not be something that you have to give. Getting others involved with different skills, ideas and relationships can all be a great way of helping reset a care system that feels like it's floundering. As much as feels right, helping the person you care for to be heard, to be involved is an amazing gift. Sometimes our health and legal systems may need a little bit of extra help to really pay attention to a person with dementia. We really thank you for all that you're doing to support clinicians (like me) know what we should be doing to provide the best care that we can.

For *clinicians and policy makers*, I'd highly recommend that we focus as much on living well with dementia as on attempts to fight dementia. Regardless of any success in changing dementia's natural history for people, we will need to be focusing on caring and creating meaning for an increasing number of people for decades in the future. I'd suggest that a systems view of dementia would encourage us to focus on supporting and empowering non-vocational carers and people with dementia themselves as key partners in figuring out what care should look like and involve. This will probably require a lot of listening and a humility from those of us who are used to telling and knowing. It's probable that a lot needs to change to improve things. Systemic reviews of the conduct of aged and dementia care in many countries including within the Australian Royal Commission into Aged Care have suggested that the potential and the necessity for improvement is great. Person-centred care practices are a good start but may become superficial in practice and remain theoretically contested. Surrogate decision-making approaches have and remain a good mechanism to make sure that we're helping people with dementia to remain safe and heard. But supported decision-making approaches and techniques can enhance or supplant surrogate decision-making and would be worthwhile for us to explore further. I'd encourage that we try to avoid seeing care for people with dementia as primarily an opportunity to express the dignity of a past person, but also to use whatever means we can muster to support that person to explore and grow through each day.

• • •

For *everyone else*, know that we've all got skin in this game. A good many of us will become carers or people with dementia at some point even if that seems a comfortably distant thought to you at this point. Regardless, the systemic nature of the dementia experience means that we can all do a lot to help or to hurt. I'd encourage you to think about how you talk about our older people and about people with dementia. I'd encourage you to wonder about what our media is influencing us towards when they tell stories about dementia, people who have the condition and dementia care. I'd encourage you to remember that dementia can be pathology, adaptation and healing all at the same time when you're talking to someone with an experience of dementia and dementia care. I'd encourage you to think, act and vote knowing that dementia will continue to impact us all and that we're all in this together.

2. An ending and a beginning

My research shared with you in this book has left us with much to consider and little in the way of conclusive answers. A fairly simple idea has been explored in a lot of different ways. This idea is that dementia isn't a single disease or pathology, it isn't even a syndrome of different pathologies, it's something more interesting and more complex. Dementia is a web of changes and responses in a host of human systems. It starts with a stone hitting the water, a set of incompletely understood neuro-biological changes in a person's brain, but the impact ripples out from there. The waves of dementia have their impact on human mental, psychological, physical, social, cultural, political, financial and language systems and these systems respond in a myriad of different ways.

Dementia isn't a brain pathology, it is all this systemic change happening continuously. I think this perspective is important for many reasons but perhaps the most important is that rethinking dementia in this way is an important seed in our efforts to improve it. This way of seeing dementia allows us the possibility of reinterpreting the experience of dementia. Dementia doesn't have to just be a terrifying descent into the monstrous or being overwhelmed by progressive pathology. What we experience as dementia could also be seen as adaptation, as a human attempt at healing and making sense of something new, un-chosen and often distressing. This way of thinking about dementia doesn't mean that it's any easier to understand or live with. It does, however, create some room for other ways of engaging with dementia. It makes some space for creativity, some space for a shared frailty and vulnerability, and some space for a hope within dementia that doesn't require someone in a lab somewhere to patent a cure. Nevertheless, let's not forget that dementia *systems*, like other systems, change on their own terms and for their own reasons. Improvements will be possible but will only emerge through the operation of complex partnerships. This way of thinking also cautions us that dementia is here to stay whatever we do, dementia has changed and is changing us. More change is inevitable but that won't turn the clock back for any of us. Dementia also teaches me about how fragile we are and how incomplete without each other. It offers an opportunity to learn more about ourselves and the world.

I've tried to provide reasoned and compassionate arguments for why we should look at dementia in this way but it's quite possible that you remain far from convinced. My hope is that together at this moment we can collectively feel some uncertainty, some kind of lingering openness and sense that there is more to dementia than we may previously have thought and read and heard. I hope that rethinking dementia in this structured and detailed way can enable the problems and experiences of dementia to be viewed in a different light. There is wisdom, sometimes, in maintaining uncertainty.

Our uncertainty also allows us to feel that there is still a need to explore and discover dementia, that we haven't got the answers yet. Accepting this uncertain position also allows dementia to remain a question and the fertile potential of this should not be underestimated. A question drives our need for examination, to think, feel and work harder in response. The philosopher, Hegel, once noted that, "The owl of Minerva takes its flight only when the shades of night are gathering" (Hegel, 1952). It is sometimes the moments and problems that pose the greatest challenge that spur the insight, wisdom and compassion of which we are capable.

Dementia remains one of the tragic challenges facing our society. However, rethinking dementia and recognising its complexity presents us with opportunities. The first is to re-examine our assumptions about what dementia means. Dementia is not just a monstrous descent, a neurobiological condition, or a disease that affects an otherwise unchanging self or person. It is not just a process that exposes changes in relationships, the co-construction of identity, and the fragility of an independent self. Dementia is "not just" the many things we think about it. It is a combination of all these things, and more, interacting together. It is something to which a vast number of factors contribute including our own responses to it. So, if we want to understand the experience of dementia, we have more work to do. Understanding dementia requires us to recognise that all of these systems and interactions contribute to what dementia is and means. Understanding dementia means recognising that it isn't a fixed and singular thing but something that is evolving and something that we all have a part in shaping.

Writing these words, I'm reminded of an experience from many years ago: I was lying on my back among some trees with my face turned toward the sun and my eyes closed. The light was bright, an intense fleshy pink beating through my eyelids. I turned my head toward the safety of the green overhead, opened my eyes and was immediately dazzled. Everything in front and around me was washed out in an incandescent white brightness. Slowly, the images resolved into trees and leaves, colours and movement, an intricate picture from the overwhelming intensity of what it had been moments before. I remembered this moment while thinking about rethinking dementia, the sense of being overwhelmed by something vast, inescapable and encompassing that can yet resolve into something human, concrete and familiar.

The intensity of the challenge of dementia feels overwhelming. Thinking through the systems that contribute to the dementia experience can also feel like we're making something huge even more complicated. But that isn't the case. All of that complexity is there already. All of that complexity is why dementia is so overwhelming in the first place. My hope is that through this shift in focus we might all see that within the complexity of dementia there's a lot that seems understandable and tangible to us. We may even start to see that there are ways that we can shift the experience of dementia right now.

The complexity of dementia, perhaps more than any other "diagnosis", means that we cannot understand all that's going on without opening our eyes to this world of underlying systems. If we were being generous, we could even say that by being so complicated, so overwhelming, so tragic and so urgent, dementia presents us with somewhat of a gift. Dementia enables us, out of sheer necessity, to better understand how we work and how our world works with us. These sorts of systems were always underlying how illnesses work and how they are experienced. They contribute to how we value our lives and what we express about ourselves and others. They're actually completely central to how we live. These systems were always there, but mostly we don't really need to pay that much attention to them. Rethinking dementia creates a challenging but important opportunity for us to learn something about ourselves. To discover ourselves as fragile, dynamic and interconnected.

We are all connected to dementia, and it to us, through systems. We, and it, rely on and persist through systems. We may be able to learn from dementia that we are more than our memories, our rationality, our physical form, or the illusion of our independence. We are reliant, inter-dependent and interconnected, mobile and embodied, fragile and yet resilient. We're connected to dementia. We share a border with it, and through this we have influence. We have the power to reinterpret dementia's meaning, to shape what we feel about people with dementia and how we treat them. We may never feel that we completely understand dementia, that we have discovered all of its mysteries. But through the energy and effort to try to understand dementia we may learn more about how we are connected to this world and each other, to its difficulties, to its responsibilities and to its capacity to change. For all that dementia has taken from us, individually and collectively, we might find that through learning and responding to its challenge we are enriched.

· · · · · ·

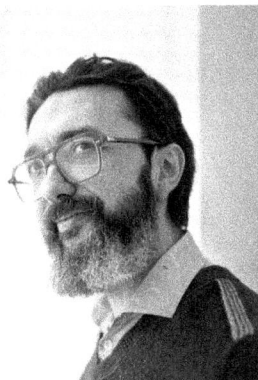

Michael Chapman is a dual specialist in geriatric and palliative medicine based at a metropolitan hospital on Ngunnawal country in Canberra, Australia. Michael's research focuses on issues of ageing, death and dying. He has a particular interest in dementia and cognitive impairment, in care ethics, and in exploring and supporting care systems. Michael has roles with multiple universities and academic journals and is the recipient of numerous project grants including from the Australian Medical Research Futures Fund.

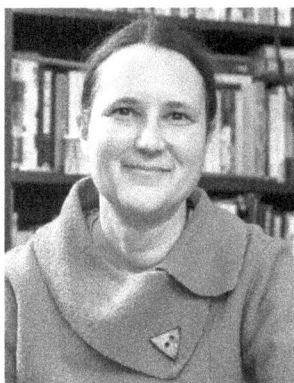

Mirranda Burton is a printmaker, animator, educator, illustrator and graphic story-teller based on Wurundjeri land, Melbourne, Australia. Her first graphic novel *Hidden* was published in 2011 by Black Pepper Publishing. Her second graphic novel *Underground: Marsupial Outlaws and Other Rebels of Australia's War in Vietnam* was released by Allen & Unwin in 2021. Both titles have been released in French by La Boîte à Bulles. www.mirrandaburton.com

Endnotes

1   This is credited to Abraham Maslow and is sometimes called the "law of the instrument".

2   The Enlightenment was a period in Europe often described as lasting from 1685 up until 1815 and including significant changes in philosophical, scientific, and political thought.

3   Kant's categorical imperative, "Act so that the maxims of thy action might become a universal law" (Kant et al., 2002: 37), provides the rational framework for moral behaviour. It suggests that an action is moral if we can formulate a statement which describes our reasons for an action, then re-frame that statement as a universal law that would apply to all rational people, consider whether this rule would be conceivable in our world governed by the laws of nature, and then ask ourselves whether we would or could rationally carry through with this rule if everyone was supposed to (Rawls, 1999).

4   Autonomy probably includes: the capacity or ability to govern ourselves (being able to be autonomous), actually doing or achieving this (being autonomous), an ideal that we find important that we might aspire to (wanting autonomy), and as a right or set of rights which expresses our self-governance (having a right to autonomy).

5   Behavioural variant fronto-temporal dementia refers to a subset of dementia which occurs in a younger age group (often people in their 50s) and is characterised primarily by changes in behaviour. Changes like apathy, lack of motivation, loss of sympathy or empathy, overeating, repetitive behaviours and impaired judgement are all common features of the condition.

6   I'm simplifying things a little here. A fuller description would acknowledge that most of what has been discussed to this point is called ethics. Specifically, it would be within a major category of ethical discussion called normative ethics (sometimes called ethical theory), which focuses on coming up with reasoned ideas about how moral choices work and what they consist of. Kant's work, for instance, is central to a highly influential branch of normative ethics called "deontology". There are two other major categories of ethics that are usually described. The first is meta-ethics which addresses whether morality exists and how to understand it, which I note here but will not be mentioning again. The second, which is going to be a big focus for the rest of this book, is applied ethics which focuses on what ethics means in real-life situations, that is, what's the best thing to do in a specific situation.

7   A topic of heightened focus during the COVID-19 pandemic with implications for debates on a variety of public health and safety measures including lockdown, mandatory vaccination, and use of PPE such as masks.

8   This has been argued as arising from a persisting and subtle exploitation of the fundamental human wish for meaning and wellbeing (Szejnwald Brown & Vergragt, 2016).

9   The Nuremberg Trials, conducted from 1945–1946, exposed the crimes of the Nazi German leadership during World War 2. Evidence of experimentation on prisoners to further military, medical and ideological goals with frequently lethal consequences was made public to a horrified world. This resulted in the development of The Nuremberg Code as a first step towards contemporary health research ethics.

10 An alarming example of unethical health research was the Tuskegee Syphilis Study which began in 1932 in the United States. In this experiment African American men were invited to participate in a study in return for additional healthcare. The study intended to examine the effects of syphilis over time, however participants weren't told they had syphilis or offered the effective treatments that were available. The study persisted for 40 years and resulted in the harm and deaths of many people. There are multiple other tragic examples of this kind of unethical research from many countries around the world.

11 The rules are a little different in emergencies as there's acceptance that if a person needs an emergency treatment there may not be time, or they may not be able to provide consent for a lifesaving treatment.

12 Much of this research is conducted or interpreted within a positivist framework, which sees the complex fluidity of real-world decision-making within a concrete, definable and "objective" perspective. This body of work frequently fails to acknowledge the complexity of the issues underlying the meaning of decision-making for persons with dementia, and yet its contributions are notable, nonetheless.

13 It is perhaps useful to note here that terminology can complicate these issues. While sometimes used interchangeably, "capacity" and "competence" are differentiated in that competence is a legal term defined by the ability (under law) to perform an action (Barbas & Wilde, 2001).

14 The rules around all of this are highly dependent on where you happen to be. If you are in Australia this website might be useful: https://end-of-life.qut.edu.au.

15 Advance care planning and its legal endorsement through advance care directives have received significant support through policy and practice as a gold-standard approach. The evidence to support their beneficial outcomes, however, remains variable and best-practice approaches to these interventions and their assessment (for all populations) will likely remain a work in progress for some time (McMahan et al., 2021).

16 As a palliative care doctor, I think it's important to add here that I'm not trying to argue that aggressive, medicalised support for people with advanced dementia is required, or beneficial. This section isn't specifically trying to explore those kinds of decisions but raises the point that listening to and hearing people with dementia in decisions related to them is important and not done often enough.

17 Even this is simplifying a complicated space and there are different ways of talking about personhood, what it means and what is important about it, but this approach seems helpful for what we're trying to explore here.

18 Tom Kitwood's highly influential book *Dementia Reconsidered* (Open University Press, 1997) was published in the 12 months prior to his untimely death in 1998. He would never know the lasting impact that he has had on thinking about dementia care.

19 Here Lindemann's imagery is also being used to explore and highlight a point from Wittgenstein's philosophy about personhood as expression and recognition.

20 Parfit discusses a thought experiment where, due to a disastrous trauma, one triplet's brain is removed, and each hemisphere is transplanted by a skilled surgeon into the damaged brains of the two remaining siblings. This fission lays bare identity's uncertainties, while allowing the possibility of psychological continuity and

connectedness. The result, for Parfit, is a situation where siblings may remember and enact the experiences and preferences of the sibling whose brain was divided, without considering themselves to be that person. Equally, if we consider one of these siblings as the original, we must consider both as that original identity, their own identities lost in the process of trying to explain the continuation of the donor sibling.

21 This is from the work of Charles Taylor, a Canadian philosopher who was particularly interested in the notion of the self.

22 Alasdair MacIntyre was a Scottish-American philosopher who was instrumental in the greater focus on Aristotelean virtue in more recent philosophy.

23 A key early work here was the Belmont Report produced in the US after a slew of troubling cases of unethical research. Many guidelines are now available to support safe research for vulnerable populations such as the NHMRC national statement on ethical conduct in research in Australia. See National Statement on Ethical Conduct in Human Research (2007) – Updated 2018 | NHMRC.

24 For a more in-depth discussion of this consider the excellent article by Carter & Little, 2007.

25 For more information on this vast topic you may wish to read this seminal work from J-F. Lyotard (Lyotard, 1979). A more contemporary view from Paul Komesaroff explores the implications for healthcare (Komesaroff, 2008a).

26 This coheres with ideas of "co-creation", "co-development" and "co-design" which are important areas of growing focus in health research.

27 Ethnography is a type of direct description of a group, culture or community which involves observation and participation in that environment over a sustained period of time (Hammersley & Atkinson, 1995).

28 See "Our, not your, dementia".

29 The behavioural and psychological symptoms of dementia (BPSD) are common complications of dementia. They can occur in up to 80% of people with the diagnosis at some point during their illness (Gauthier 2010). There are a lot of different types of symptoms in this syndrome including wandering, calling out, mood changes, aggression and many others. BPSD is (more than dementia itself) often understood as more than just a neurobiological problem and the effects of environment; and care behaviours are understood as often having an impact on the symptoms and severity of the problems. (See Gauthier, S., Cummings, J., Ballard, C., Brodaty, H., Grossberg, G., Robert, P., & Lyketsos, C. (2010). "Management of behavioural problems in Alzheimer's disease". *International Psychogeriatrics / IPA*, 22(3), 346–372. https://doi.org/10.1017/S1041610209991505.

30 As a palliative care doctor, I'd be hesitant to suggest that dying from dementia is a "good" or "bad" way to die. Any process of dying can be good or bad and there are many factors beyond the condition that a person's dying from which influence these things. Jenny Van Der Steen has written a lot about what tends to happen when a person with dementia is getting close to dying; and the European Association of Palliative Care White Paper on palliative care in dementia discusses what good care should include. This paper from Frank Brennan and others including myself summarises some of what this means in an Australian context: Brennan, F., Chapman, M., Gardiner, M. D., Narasimhan, M., & Cohen, J. (2023). "Our dementia challenge: Arise palliative care". *Internal Medicine Journal*, 53(2), 186–193. https://doi.org/10.1111/imj.16011.

31 These sorts of small decisions are akin to decisions about experiential interest discussed by Dresser and Dworkin. Dworkin felt these are less important than critical decisions which he also felt people with dementia were not validly able to decide about. Dresser argued that these are actually central to our experience, and arguably even more important for people with dementia (Dresser, 1995).

32 Which we might be able to refer to as an internal influence or compulsion based on Dubljevic's descriptions (Dubljevic, 2013).

33 This is a scientific term that refers to the way an object appears in a different position when you view it from different points.

34 From Borges' story *The Garden of Forking Paths* where the choices that we make have multiple different impacts and relevance, some more apparent than others.

35 See previous section "The weight of dementia".

36 See "Stepping stones in the river".

37 Additionally, there have been many highly important contributors to systems thinking and it is an area, like all areas of science, were debate and work continues. For simplicity I will continue to refer to a variety of ideas within the broad church of systems work as systems theory or systems thinking, while acknowledging that there are a number of critical areas of work that contribute to this space not limited to work on complexity science and complex adaptive systems.

38 In using this example I'm consciously not elaborating on how my immune system and neuromuscular system are part of one system, that is, the system that collects all the systems that make up me, the system that is Michael Chapman. One of the tricky things about systems thinking is that systems are so central to how things are that there's always another level. It is (to misquote Bertrand Russell) "systems all the way down".

39 The phrase refers to a geometry problem where someone (not me) might try to construct a square with the area of a circle using geometrical tools.

40 There is also a further relegation of the participation and value of people with dementia from an increasing focus on the importance of our connected, "liquid modern" identities in social media. They risk being effectively excluded from modes of exploration which, regardless of the outcomes for those involved, are now considered important and self-defining.

41 This has been explored in many media and academic articles. A recent examination of writing on Facebook highlighted the fear that many people feel about dying with dementia and the hope that legal changes including VAD access may provide some alternative (Dehkhoda, 2020).

42 There have been many different ways of defending this seemingly pretty obvious point that people have worth. Historically, religion was central to this, though a number of non-religious schools of thought, like humanism, have sought to defend the importance of people in themselves without seeking to say they're important or valuable because of their relationship to a higher power or set of inviolable rules.

43 A valid question in response to this view of experience would be: if that is true, is there anything that is singular and mine, that is, not dependent on all of these systems? Many have argued that even our most basic constant and almost always unconscious sense of being alive in our bodies arises from interaction between parts of our brain and our bodies (Fuchs 2017). It seems we have always been a collection of interactive processes for as long as we've been us.

44 This is Varela's term implying that our minds are just as embedded in and connected to the world being experienced as compared with the brain and mind observing and interpreting a world "around" us.

45 This distinction comes from Maturana's noting that because all systems self-define their responses to what they receive there is no such thing as pure information as it will always be subject to the interpretation of the system that's trying to make sense of it.

46 For a distressing account of this issue in the Australian context, the Royal Commission into Aged Care is recommended and harrowing reading.

• • •

Bibliography

Adams, T., & Gardiner, P. (2005). "Communication and interaction within dementia care triads: Developing a theory for relationship-centred care". *Dementia*, *4*(2), 185–205. https://doi.org/10.1177/1471301205051092

Agich, G. J. (1993a). "A phenomenological view of social action". In *Autonomy and Long-Term Care* (pp. 114–153). Oxford University Press.

Agich, G. J. (1993b). *Autonomy and long-term care*. Oxford University Press.

Agich, G. J. (2003). *Dependence and Autonomy in Old Age: An Ethical Framework for Long-Term Care Second and Revised Edition*. Cambridge University Press.

Alexander, G. C., Emerson, S., & Kesselheim, A. S. (2021). "Evaluation of Aducanumab for Alzheimer Disease: Scientific Evidence and Regulatory Review Involving Efficacy, Safety, and Futility". *JAMA - Journal of the American Medical Association*, *325*(17), 1717–1718. https://doi.org/10.1001/JAMA.2021.3854

Andersen, C. (2019). "Exploring Aboriginal Identity in Australia and Building Resilience". In L. Klain-Gabbay (Ed.), *Indigenous, Aboriginal, Fugitive and Ethnic Groups Around the Globe*. IntechOpen. https://doi.org/10.5772/intechopen.86677

Apostolova, L. G. (2016). "Alzheimer Disease". *Continuum: Lifelong Learning in Neurology*, *22*(2 Dementia), 419–434. https://doi.org/10.1212/CON.0000000000000307

Armstrong, K., Schwartz, J. S., & Fitzgerald, G. (2002). "Effect of framing as gain versus loss on understanding and hypothetical treatment choices: Survival and mortality curves". *Medical Decision Making*, *22*(1), 76–83.

Ashley, V. (2012). "The Essex Autonomy Project Green Paper Technical Report Philosophical Models of Personal Autonomy". In *Essex Autonomy Project Green Paper Report* (192). University of Essex: Essex Autonomy Project.

Azétsop, J., & Rennie, S. (2010). "Principlism, medical individualism, and health promotion in resource-poor countries: Can autonomy-based bioethics promote social justice and population health?" *Philosophy, Ethics, and Humanities in Medicine: PEHM*, *5*, 1. https://doi.org/10.1186/1747-5341-5-1

Badrakalimuthu, V., & Barclay, S. (2014). "Do people with dementia die at their preferred location of death? A systematic literature review and narrative synthesis". *Age and Ageing*, *43*(1), 13–19. https://doi.org/10.1093/ageing/aft151

Baier, Annette. (1985). *Postures of the mind: Essays on mind and morals*. Methuen.

Bailly, Lionel. (2009). *Lacan: A beginner's guide*. Oneworld. https://books.google.com.au/books/about/Lacan.html?id=S0vuAAAAMAAJ&redir_esc=y

Barbas, N. R., & Wilde, E. A. (2001). "Competency issues in dementia: Medical decision making, driving, and independent living". *Journal of Geriatric Psychiatry and Neurology*, *14*(4), 199–212. https://doi.org/10.1177/089198870101400405

Barker, P., & Chang, J. (2013). "Complex Problems and Second-Order Change". In *Basic Family Therapy* (pp. 147–171). John Wiley & Sons Ltd. https://doi.org/10.1002/9781118624944.ch11

Bartlett, R., Gjernes, T., Lotherington, A. T., & Obstefelder, A. (2018). "Gender, citizenship and dementia care: A scoping review of studies to inform policy and future research". In *Health and Social Care in the Community*. https://doi.org/10.1111/hsc.12340

Bartlett, R., & O'Connor, D. (2007). "From personhood to citizenship: Broadening the lens for dementia practice and research". *Journal Of Aging Studies*, *21*(2), 107–118. https://doi.org/10.1016/j.jaging.2006.09.002

Bateman, Chris. (2014). *Chaos Ethics*. John Hunt Publishing.

Bateson, G. (1972a). *Steps to an Ecology of Mind: Collected Essays in Anthropology, Psychiatry, Evolution, and Epistemology*. Ballantine Books. http://www.abebooks.com/servlet/BookDetailsPL?bi=7457332430&searchurl=curl=/isbn/0345273702/

Bateson, G. (1972b). "The cybernetics of 'self': A theory of alcoholism". In *Steps to an ecology of mind: Collated essays in anthropology, psychiatry, evolution and epistemology*. (pp. 309–337). Ballantine Books.

Bauman, Z. (2004a). "Identity". In *Identity: Conversations with Benedetto Vecchi* (pp. 9–99).

Bauman, Z. (2004b). *Identity: Conversations With Benedetto Vecchi*. Wiley. https://books.google.com/books/about/Identity.html?id=xkA_0mmQcloC&pgis=1

Bauman, Z., & May, T. (2001). *Thinking sociologically*. Blackwell Publishers.

Beauchamp, T., & Childress, J. (1994). *Principles of biomedical ethics* (4th ed.). Oxford University Press.

Beauchamp, T. L. (1999). "The failure of theories of personhood". *Kennedy Institute of Ethics Journal*, *9.4*, 309–324.

Beauchamp, T. L. (2005). *Who deserves autonomy, and whose autonomy deserves respect*? http://philpapers.org/rec/BEAWDA

Beecher, H. K. (1966). "Ethics and clinical research". *New England Journal of Medicine*, *274*, 1354–1360.

Behuniak, S. M. (2010). "Toward a political model of dementia: Power as compassionate care". *Journal of Aging Studies*, *24*(4), 231–240. https://doi.org/10.1016/j.jaging.2010.05.003

Behuniak, S. M. (2011). "The living dead? The construction of people with Alzheimer's disease as zombies". *Ageing and Society*, *31*(01), 70–92. https://doi.org/10.1017/S0144686X10000693

Bérubé, M. (1996). *Life as We Know it: A Father, a Family, and an Exceptional Child*. Pantheon Books. https://books.google.com.au/books/about/Life_as_We_Know_it.html?id=buskAAAAYAAJ&pgis=1

Bleakley, A., Marshall, R., & Levine, D. (2014). "He drove forward with a yell: Anger in medicine and Homer". *Medical Humanities*, *40*, 22–30. https://doi.org/10.1136/medhum-2013-010432

Bohman, J., & Rehg, W. (2007). *Jürgen Habermas*. http://plato.stanford.edu/entries/habermas/#TheComAct

Boulding, K., & Khalil, E. (2002). *Evolution, Order and Complexity*. Routledge. http://books.google.com/books?hl=en&lr=&id=hPmEAgAAQBAJ&pgis=1

Bowman, D. (2008). "Who decides who decides? Ethical perspectives on capacity and decision-making". In G. Stoppe (Ed.), *Competence assessment in dementia*. (pp. 51–59). Springer Publishing Co. https://doi.org/10.1007/978-3-211-72369-2_6

Brady, V. (1994). *Caught in the draught: Essays on Contemporary Australian Society and Culture*. HarperCollins Publishers.

Brijnath, B., & Manderson, L. (2008). "Discipline in chaos: Foucault, dementia and aging in India". *Culture, Medicine and Psychiatry*, *32*(4), 607–626. https://doi.org/10.1007/s11013-008-9111-5

Brison, S. (2000). "Relational autonomy and freedom of expression". In Catriona. Mackenzie & N. Stoljar (Eds.), *Relational Autonomy: Feminist Perspectives on Autonomy, Agency, and the Social Self*. OUP Oxford. http://philpapers.org/rec/BRIRAA-5

Bristow, W. (2010). *Enlightenment*. Stanford Encyclopedia of Philosophy. https://plato.stanford.edu/entries/enlightenment/

Brooker, D. (2004). "What is person-centred care in dementia?" *Reviews in Clinical Gerontology*, *13*(03), 215–222. https://doi.org/10.1017/s095925980400108x

Brookes, G., Harvey, K., Chadborn, N., & Dening, T. (2018). "'Our biggest killer': Multimodal discourse representations of dementia in the British press". *Social Semiotics*, *28*(3), 371–395. https://doi.org/10.1080/10350330.2017.1345111

Burke, L. (2007). *Alzheimer's Disease: Personhood and first person testimony* (Vol. 2013, Issue 26/06). www.cdsrn.org.uk/Burke_CDSRN_2007.pdf

Burke, L. (2014). "Oneself as Another: Intersubjectivity and Ethics in Alzheimer's Illness Narratives". *Narrative Works: Issues, Investigations & Interventions*, *4*(2), 28–47.

Burke, L. (2016). *The Fear: Popular representations of dementia and the logic of disaster capitalism* (pp. 1–10). University of Warwick.

Burks, H. B., des Bordes, J. K. A., Chadha, R., Holmes, H. M., & Rianon, N. J. (2021). "Quality of Life Assessment in Older Adults with Dementia: A Systematic Review". *Dementia and Geriatric Cognitive Disorders*, *50*(2), 103–110. https://doi.org/10.1159/000515317

Burr, V. (1995). *An Introduction to Social Constructionism*. Routledge. http://books.google.com.au/books?id=7du5229Pc4EC

Campbell, A. V. (2003). "The virtues (and vices) of the four principles". *Journal of Medical Ethics*, *29*(5), 292–296. https://doi.org/10.1136/jme.29.5.292

Carter, S. M., & Little, M. (2007). "Justifying knowledge, justifying method, taking action: Epistemologies, methodologies, and methods in qualitative research". *Qualitative Health Research*, *17*(10), 1316–1328. https://doi.org/10.1177/1049732307306927

Castells, M. (1997). *The power of identity*. Blackwell. http://dl.acm.org/citation.cfm?id=523266

Castoriadis, C. (1991). "Power, Politics, Autonomy". In *Philosophy, Politics, Autonomy*. Oxford University Press.

Chapman, M., Philip, J., Gardner, S., & Komesaroff, P. (2019). "Fragile objects: A visual essay". *Journal of Bioethical Inquiry*, *16*(2). https://doi.org/10.1007/s11673-019-09911-7

Chapman, M., Philip, J., & Komesaroff, P. (2018). "Making Sense of Senselessness: Contemporary Literary Commentaries on Dementia". *OBM Geriatrics*, *3*(2), 1–1. https://doi.org/10.21926/obm.geriatr.1902056

Chapman, M., Philip, J., & Komesaroff, P. (2022). "A person-centred problem". *Humanities and Social Sciences Communications 9*, *154*. https://doi.org/10.1057/s41599-022-01166-9

Charon, R. (2006). *Narrative Medicine*. Oxford University Press. https://global.oup.com/academic/product/narrative-medicine-9780195340228?cc=au&lang=en&

Chattopadhyay, S., & De Vries, R. (2008). "Bioethical concerns are global, bioethics is Western". *Eubios Journal of Asian and International Bioethics: EJAIB*, *18*(4), 106–109.

Chrisp, T. A. C., Tabberer, S., & Thomas, B. D. (2013). "Bounded autonomy in deciding to seek medical help: Carer role, the sick role and the case of dementia". *Journal of Health Psychology*, *18*(2), 272–281. https://doi.org/10.1177/1359105312437265

Christman, J. (1989). "Introduction". In J. Christman (Ed.), *The Inner Citadel: Essays on individual autonomy*. Oxford University Press.

Christman, J. (2020). *Autonomy in moral and political philosophy*. Stanford Encyclopedia of Philosophy. https://plato.stanford.edu/entries/autonomy-moral/

Clouser, K. D., & Gert, B. (1990). "A critique of principlism". *The Journal of Medicine and Philosophy*, *15*, 219–236. https://doi.org/10.1093/jmp/15.2.219

Coetzee, R. H., Leask, S. J., & Jones, R. G. (2003). "The attitudes of carers and old age psychiatrists towards the treatment of potentially fatal events in end-stage dementia". *International Journal of Geriatric Psychiatry*, *18*(2), 169–173.

Collier, A., & Chapman, M. (2023). "Matters of care and the good death—Rhetoric or reality?" *Current Opinion in Supportive and Palliative Care*, 17(3), 208–213. https://doi.org/10.1097/SPC.0000000000000663

Congedo, M., Causarano, R. I., Alberti, F., Bonito, V., Borghi, L., Colombi, L., Defanti, C. A., Marcello, N., Porteri, C., Pucci, E., Tarquini, D., Tettamanti, M., Tiezzi, A., Tiraboschi, P., & Gasparini, M. (2010). "Ethical issues in end-of-life treatments for patients with dementia". *European Journal Of Neurology: The Official Journal Of The European Federation Of Neurological Societies*, *17*(6), 774–779. https://doi.org/10.1111/j.1468-1331.2010.02991.x

Couteur, D., Doust, J., Creasey, H., & Brayne, C. (2013). "Political drive to screen for pre-dementia: Not evidence based and ignores the harms of diagnosis". *BMJ: British Medical Journal*, *5125*(September), 1–6. https://doi.org/10.1136/bmj.f5125

Cummings, J. L., Morstorf, T., & Zhong, K. (2014). "Alzheimer's disease drug-development pipeline: Few candidates, frequent failures". *Alzheimer's Research & Therapy*, *6*, 37. https://doi.org/10.1186/alzrt269

Darzins, P., & Molloy, W. (2000). *Who Can Decide?: The Six Step Capacity Assessment Process*. Memory Australia Press. https://books.google.com.au/books/about/Who_Can_Decide.html?id=6tvYAAAACAAJ&pgis=1

de Boer, M. E., Hertogh, C. M. P. M., Dröes, R.-M., Jonker, C., & Eefsting, J. A. (2010). "Advance directives in dementia: Issues of validity and effectiveness". *International Psychogeriatrics / IPA*, *22*, 201–208. https://doi.org/10.1017/S1041610209990706

de Spinoza, B. (2001). *Ethics*. Wordsworth Editions. https://books.google.com.au/books/about/Ethics.html?id=FJrOf7k44NMC&redir_esc=y

Dehkhoda, A., Owens, R. G., & Malpas, P. J. (2020). "A Netnographic Approach: Views on Assisted Dying for Individuals with Dementia". *Qualitative Health Research*, 30(13), 2077–2091. https://doi.org/10.1177/1049732320925795

Degrazia, D. (2005). *Human Identity and Bioethics*. Cambridge University Press. www.cambridge.org

Delazer, M., Sinz, H., Zamarian, L., & Benke, T. (2007). "Decision-making with explicit and stable rules in mild Alzheimer's disease". *Neuropsychologia*, *45*(8), 1632–1641.

Deleuze, G., Guattari, P., & Guattari, F. (1987). "A thousand plateaus: Capitalism and schizophrenia". In *Writing* (Vol. 19). https://doi.org/10.1017/CCO9780511753657.008

Dell, P. F. (1985). "Understanding Bateson and Maturana: Toward a Biological Foundation for the Social Sciences". *Journal of Marital and Family Therapy*, *11*(1), 1–20. https://doi.org/10.1111/j.1752-0606.1985.tb00587.x

Deture, M. A., & Dickson, D. W. (2019). "The neuropathological diagnosis of Alzheimer's disease". *Molecular Neurodegeneration, 14*(1), 1–18. https://doi.org/10.1186/s13024-019-0333-5

Dewing, J. (2008a). "Personhood and dementia: Revisiting Tom Kitwood's ideas". *International Journal of Older People Nursing, 3*(1), 3–13. https://doi.org/10.1111/j.1748-3743.2007.00103.x

Dewing, J. (2008b). "Process Consent and Research with Older Persons Living with Dementia". *Research Ethics, 4*(2), 59–64. https://doi.org/10.1177/174701610800400205

Donchin, A. (2000). "Autonomy, interdependence, and assisted suicide: Respecting boundaries/crossing lines". *Bioethics, 14*(3), 187–204.

Donchin, A. (2001). "Understanding autonomy relationally: Towards a reconfiguration of bioethical principles". *Journal of Medicine and Philosophy, 26*(4).

Doyle, C. J., Dunt, D. R., Pirkis, J., Dare, A., Day, S., & Wijesundara, B. S. (2012). "Media reports on dementia: Quality and type of messages in Australian media". *Australasian Journal on Ageing, 31*(2), 96–101. https://doi.org/10.1111/j.1741-6612.2011.00543.x

Dresser, R. (1995). "Dworkin on dementia: Elegant theory, questionable policy". *The Hastings Center Report, 25*(6), 32–38.

Dubljevic, V. (2013). "Autonomy in Neuroethics: Political and Not Metaphysical". *AJOB Neuroscience, 4*(4). https://doi.org/10.1080/21507740.2013.819390

Dubljevic, V. (2020). "The Principle of Autonomy and Behavioural Variant Frontotemporal Dementia". *Bioethical Inquiry, 17*, 271–282. https://doi.org/10.1007/s11673-020-09972-z

Dunn, B., Stein, P., & Cavazzoni, P. (2021). "Approval of Aducanumab for Alzheimer Disease: The FDA's Perspective". *JAMA Internal Medicine.* https://doi.org/10.1001/jamainternmed.2021.4607

Dworkin, G. (1976). "Autonomy and behavior control". *The Hastings Center Report, 6*(1), 23–28.

Dworkin, R. (1993). *Life's Dominion: An Argument about Abortion, Euthanasia, and Individual Freedom.* Knopf. https://books.google.com.au/books/about/Life_s_Dominion.html?id=u4gp6Le3EbYC&pgis=1

Edvardsson, D., Winblad, B., & Sandman, P. (2008). "Person-centred care of people with severe Alzheimer's disease: Current status and ways forward". *The Lancet Neurology, 7*(4), 362–367. https://doi.org/10.1016/S1474-4422(08)70063-2

Ekstrom, L. W. (1993). "A Coherence Theory of Autonomy". *Philosophy and Phenomenological Research, 53*(3), 599. https://doi.org/10.2307/2108082

Elliott, B. A., Gessert, C. E., & Peden-McAlpine, C. (2007). "Decision making on behalf of elders with advanced cognitive impairment: Family transitions". *Alzheimer Disease and Associated Disorders, 21*(1), 49–54. https://doi.org/10.1097/WAD.0b013e318030840a

Elliott, C. (1999). *Bioethics, culture and identity: A philosophical disease.* Routledge.

Ely, Margot., Vinz, R., Downing, M., & Anzul, M. (1997). "What is there about writing?" In *On writing qualitative research: Living by words* (pp. 7–9). RoutledgeFalmer.

Fazel, S., Hope, T., & Jacoby, R. (2000). "Effect of cognitive impairment and premorbid intelligence on treatment preferences for life-sustaining medical therapy". *The American Journal Of Psychiatry, 157*(6), 1009–1011. https://doi.org/10.1176/appi.ajp.157.6.1009

Feinberg, J. (1989). "Autonomy". In J. Christman (Ed.), *The inner citadel: Essays on individual autonomy* (pp. 27–53). Oxford University Press.

Feinberg, L. F., & Whitlatch, C. J. (2001). "Are persons with cognitive impairment able to state consistent choices?" *The Gerontologist, 41*(3), 374–382. https://doi.org/10.1093/geront/41.3.374

Felson, G., & Reiner, P. B. (2011). "How the Neuroscience of Decision Making Informs Our Conception of Autonomy". *AJOB Neuroscience, 2*(3), 3–14. http://dx.doi.org/10.1080/21507740.2011.580489

Fetherstonhaugh, D., Tarzia, L., & Nay, R. (2013). "Being central to decision making means I am still here!: The essence of decision making for people with dementia". *Journal Of Aging Studies, 27*(2), 143–150. https://doi.org/10.1016/j.jaging.2012.12.007

Fink, H. A., Linskens, E. J., Silverman, P. C., McCarten, J. R., Hemmy, L. S., Ouellette, J. M., Greer, N. L., Wilt, T. J., & Butler, M. (2020). "Accuracy of biomarker testing for neuropathologically defined Alzheimer disease in older adults with dementia: A systematic review". *Annals of Internal Medicine, 172*(10), 669–677. https://doi.org/10.7326/M19-3888

Finlayson, J. G. (2005). *Habermas: A Very Short Introduction*. OUP Oxford. https://books.google.com/books?id=ydf-9hbeh-IC&pgis=1

Fleischer, T. E. (1999). "The personhood wars". *Theoretical Medicine and Bioethics, 20*, 309–318.

Forbes, S., Bern-Klug, M., & Gessert, C. (2000). "End-of-life decision making for nursing home residents with dementia". *Journal of Nursing Scholarship: An Official Publication of Sigma Theta Tau International Honor Society of Nursing / Sigma Theta Tau, 32*(3), 251–258. https://doi.org/10.1111/j.1547-5069.2000.00251.x

Fortinsky, R. H. (2001). "Health care triads and dementia care: Integrative framework and future directions". *Aging & Mental Health, 5*(sup1), 35–48. https://doi.org/10.1080/713649999

Foucault, M. (1978). "The History of Sexuality Volume 1: An Introduction". In *Power Knowledge* (Vol. 1). Pantheon Books. https://doi.org/10.2307/1904618

Foucault, M. (1982). "The Subject and Power". *Critical Inquiry, 8*(4), 777. https://doi.org/10.1086/448181

Foucault, M. (2012). *The History of Sexuality: Vol. I.* Pantheon Books. https://doi.org/papers3://publication/doi/10.1007/978-3-540-38918-7_5459

Frank, A. W. (1995). *The wounded storyteller: Body, illness and ethics*. University of Chicago Press.

Frank, A. W. (2010a). *Letting Stories Breathe: A Socio-Narratology* (Vol. 15). University of Chicago Press. https://books.google.com.au/books/about/Letting_Stories_Breathe.html?id=fY_3X9VWhJcC&pgis=1

Frank, A. W. (2010b). *Letting Stories Breathe: A Socio-Narratology: A Socio-Narratology*. University of Chicago Press. http://books.google.com.au/books?id=fY_3X9VWh-JcC

Frankfurt, H. G. (1971). "Freedom of the Will and the Concept of a Person". *The Journal of Philosophy, 68*(1), 5–20. https://doi.org/10.2307/2024717

Franz, C. E., Barker, J. C., Kravitz, R. L., Flores, Y., Krishnan, S., & Hinton, L. (2007). "Nonmedical influences on the use of cholinesterase inhibitors in dementia care". *Alzheimer Disease and Associated Disorders, 21*(3), 241–248.

Franzen, J. (2010). *The Corrections*. HarperCollins Publishers. http://books.google.com.au/books?id=ej4hkS1dZMEC

Fraser, J. S. (2007). "How does therapy work?" In *Second order change in psychotherapy the golden thread that unites effective treatments* (pp. 1–5). American Psychological Association.

Frey, R. (2005). "Autonomy, diminished life, and the threshold for use". *Personal Autonomy: New Essays on Personal \ldots*. https://scholar.google.com/scholar?q=autonomy%2C+diminished+life+and+the+threshold+for+use&btnG=&hl=en&as_sdt=0%2C5#0

Friedman, M. (2003). *Autonomy, Gender, Politics*. Oxford University Press, USA. https://books.google.com.au/books/about/Autonomy_Gender_Politics.html?id=nm49z8LIqDcC&pgis=1

Fuchs, T. (2012). "Chapter 1". *The phenomenology of body memory*. January 2012, 9–22. https://doi.org/10.1075/aicr.84.03fuc

Fuchs, T. (2017). *Ecology of the brain: The phenomenology and biology of the embodied mind*. OUP Oxford.

Fuchs, T. (2020). "Embodiment and personal identity in dementia". *Medicine, Health Care and Philosophy, 23*. https://doi.org/10.1007/s11019-020-09973-0

Gadamer, H.-G., Weinsheimer, J., & Marshall, D. G. (1975). *Truth and Method* (Second rev). Continuum.

Gallagher, P., & Clark, K. (2002). "The ethics of surgery in the elderly demented patient with bowel obstruction". *Journal Of Medical Ethics, 28*(2), 105–108.

Genova, L. (2009). *Still Alice*. Pocket Books. http://books.google.com.au/books?id=2P-k6AWAOcJoC

George, D. R. (2010). "Overcoming the social death of dementia through language". *The Lancet, 376*.

George, D. R., & Whitehouse, P. J. (2014). "The War (on Terror) on Alzheimer's". *Dementia (London), 13*(1), 120–130. https://doi.org/10.1177/1471301212451382

George, D. R., Whitehouse, P. J., & Ballenger, J. (2011). "The Evolving Classification of Dementia: Placing the DSM-V in a Meaningful Historical and Cultural Context and Pondering the Future of 'Alzheimer's'". *Culture, Medicine, and Psychiatry, 35*(3), 417–435. https://doi.org/10.1007/s11013-011-9219-x

Germain, A., Mayland, C. R., & Jack, B. A. (2016). "The potential therapeutic value for bereaved relatives participating in research: An exploratory study". *Palliative and Supportive Care, 14*(5), 479–487. https://doi.org/10.1017/S1478951515001194

Gershon, I. (2005). "Seeing like a system". *Anthropological Theory, 5*(2), 99–116.

Gessert, C. E., Forbes, S., & Bern-Klug, M. (2000). "Planning end-of-life care for patients with dementia: Roles of families and health professionals". *Omega, 42*(4), 273–291.

Gharajedaghi, J., & Ackoff, R. L. (1984). "Mechanisms, organisms and social systems". *Strategic Management Journal, 5*(3), 289–300. https://doi.org/10.1002/smj.4250050308

Gibson, B., & Boiko, O. (2012). "Luhmann's social systems theory, health and illness". In G. Scrambler (Ed.), *Contemporary theorists for medical sociology*. Taylor & Francis.

Gill, T. M., Gahbauer, E. A., Han, L., & Allore, H. G. (2010). "Trajectories of disability in the last year of life". *New England Journal of Medicine, 362*(13), 1173–1180.

Gillon, R. (2003a). "Ethics needs principles–four can encompass the rest–and respect for autonomy should be 'first among equals'". *Journal of Medical Ethics, 29*(5), 307–312. https://doi.org/10.1136/JME.29.5.307

Gillon, R. (2003b). "Four Scenarios". *Journal of Medical Ethics, 29*, 267–268. https://doi.org/10.1136/jme.27.1.54

Givens, J. L., Kiely, D. K., Carey, K., & Mitchell, S. L. (2009). "Healthcare proxies of nursing home residents with advanced dementia: Decisions they confront and their satisfaction with decision-making". *Journal of the American Geriatrics Society, 57*(7), 1149–1155. https://doi.org/10.1111/j.1532-5415.2009.02304.x

Gleckman, H. (2012). "The Obama Administration's War on Alzheimer's". In *Forbes*. http://www.forbes.com/sites/howardgleckman/2012/01/11/the-obama-administrations-war-on-alzheimers/#13ef533deb74

Gomez-Virseda, C., de Maeseneer, Y., & Gastmans, C. (2019). "Relational autonomy: What does it mean and how is it used in end-of-life care? A systematic review of argument-based ethics literature". *BMC Medical Ethics, 20*(76). https://doi.org/10.1186/s12910-019-0417-3

Grieves, V. (2014). "Culture, not colour, is the heart of Aboriginal identity". In *The Conversation*. http://theconversation.com/culture-not-colour-is-the-heart-of-aboriginal-identity-30102

Ha, J., Kim, E.-J., Lim, S., Shin, D.-W., Kang, Y.-J., Bae, S.-M., Yoon, H.-K., & Oh, K.-S. (2012). "Altered risk-aversion and risk-taking behaviour in patients with Alzheimer's disease". *Psychogeriatrics: The Official Journal of The Japanese Psychogeriatric Society, 12*(3), 151–158. https://doi.org/10.1111/j.1479-8301.2011.00396.x

Habermas, J. (1981). "Modernity versus Postmodernity". *New German Critique, 22*, 3–14.

Habermas, J. (1990). "The Theory of Communicative Action: Vol. 2: Lifeworld and System: A Critique of Functionalist Reason". In T. McCarthy (Trans.), *Contemporary Sociology* (Vol. 19). https://doi.org/10.2307/2072540

Hamann, J., Bronner, K., Margull, J., Mendel, R., Diehl   Schmid, J., Bühner, M., Klein, R., Schneider, A., Kurz, A., & Perneczky, R. (2011). "Patient participation in medical and social decisions in Alzheimer's disease". *Journal of The American Geriatrics Society, 59*(11), 2045–2052. https://doi.org/10.1111/j.1532-5415.2011.03661.x

Hammersley, M., & Atkinson, P. (1995). *Ethnography: Principles in practice* (2nd ed.). Tavistock.

Haraway, D. J. (1991). "A Cyborg Manifesto: Science, Technology, and Socialist-Feminism in the Late Twentieth Century". In *Simians, Cyborgs and women: The reinvention of nature* (pp. 149–182). Routledge.

Haraway, D. J. (2015). *Simians, Cyborgs, and Women The Reinvention of Nature*. Routledge.

Hargreaves, Andy. (2003). *Teaching in the knowledge society: Education in the age of insecurity*. Teachers College Press.

Harrigan, M., & Gillett, G. (2009). "Hunting good will in the wilderness". In D. O'Connor & B. A. Purves (Eds.), *Decision-Making, Personhood and Dementia: Exploring the Interface*. Jessica Kingsley Publishers. https://books.google.com.au/books?hl=en&lr=&id=bQIQBQAAQBAJ&oi=fnd&pg=PA47&dq=hunting+good+will+in+the+wilderness+harrigan&ots=bplNboubzK&sig=mxY-W1A1e9KaYTgaq-FIwJmoXL7I

Hauber, A. B., Johnson, F. R., Fillit, H., Mohamed, A. F., Leibman, C., Arrighi, H. M., Grundman, M., & Townsend, R. J. (2009). "Older Americans' risk-benefit preferences for modifying the course of Alzheimer disease". *Alzheimer Disease and Associated Disorders, 23*(1), 23–32. https://doi.org/10.1097/WAD.0b013e318181e4c7

Healy, T. C. (2000). "Community-dwelling cognitively impaired frail elders: An analysis of social workers' decisions concerning support for autonomy". *Social Work In Health Care*, *30*(2), 27–47. https://doi.org/10.1300/J010v30n02_02

Hegel, G. W. F. (1952). *Philosophy of Right*. Clarendon Press. https://doi.org/10.1002/9781444354256

Helton, M. R., Cohen, L. W., Zimmerman, S., & van der Steen, J. T. (2011). "The importance of physician presence in nursing homes for residents with dementia and pneumonia". *Journal Of The American Medical Directors Association*, *12*(1), 68–73. https://doi.org/10.1016/j.jamda.2010.01.005

Helton, M. R., van der Steen, J. T., Daaleman, T. P., Gamble, G. R., & Ribbe, M. W. (2006). "A cross-cultural study of physician treatment decisions for demented nursing home patients who develop pneumonia". *Annals Of Family Medicine*, *4*(3), 221–227.

Hennelly, N., Cooney, A., Houghton, C., & O'Shea, E. (2021). "Personhood and Dementia Care: A Qualitative Evidence Synthesis of the Perspectives of People with Dementia". *Gerontologist*, *61*(3), E85–E100. https://doi.org/10.1093/geront/gnz159

Hennings, J., Froggatt, K., & Keady, J. (2010). "Approaching the end of life and dying with dementia in care homes: The accounts of family carers". *Reviews in Clinical Gerontology*, *20*(2), 114–127. https://doi.org/10.1017/S0959259810000092

Herskovits, E. (1995). "Struggling over subjectivity: Debates about 'self' and Alzheimer's disease". *Medical Anthropology Quarterly*, *9*(2), 146–164.

Higgs, P., & Gilleard, C. (2016). "Interrogating personhood and dementia". *Aging and Mental Health*, *20*(8), 773–780. https://doi.org/10.1080/13607863.2015.1118012

High, D. M. (1992). "Research with Alzheimer's disease subjects: Informed consent and proxy decision making". *Journal of The American Geriatrics Society*, *40*(9), 950–957.

Hinkka, H., Kosunen, E., Lammi, U. K., Metsänoja, R., Puustelli, A., & Kellokumpu-Lehtinen, P. (2002). "Decision making in terminal care: A survey of Finnish doctors' treatment decisions in end-of-life scenarios involving a terminal cancer and a terminal dementia patient". *Palliative Medicine*, *16*(3), 195–204. https://doi.org/10.1191/0269216302pm510oa

Hirschman, K. B., Joyce, C. M., James, B. D., Xie, S. X., & Karlawish, J. H. T. (2005). "Do Alzheimer's disease patients want to participate in a treatment decision, and would their caregivers let them?" *The Gerontologist*, *45*(3), 381–388.

Hirschman, K. B., Xie, S. X., Feudtner, C., & Karlawish, J. H. T. (2004). "How Does an Alzheimer's Disease Patient's Role in Medical Decision-Making Change Over Time?" *Journal Of Geriatric Psychiatry and Neurology*, *17*(2), 55–60. https://doi.org/10.1177/0891988704264540

Holland, E. W. (2013). *Deleuze and Guattari's A thousand plateaus: A reader's guide*.

Huthwaite, J. S., Martin, R. C., Griffith, H. R., Anderson, B., Harrell, L. E., & Marson, D. C. (2006). "Declining medical decision-making capacity in mild AD: a two-year longitudinal study". *Behavioral Sciences & The Law*, *24*(4), 453–463.

Irigaray, L. (1985). *Speculum of the other woman*. Cornell University Press.

Jaworska, A. (1999). "Respecting the Margins of Agency: Alzheimer's Patients and the Capacity to Value". *Philosophy & Public Affairs*, *28*(2), 105–138. https://doi.org/10.1111/j.1088-4963.1999.00105.x

Jaworska, A. (2004). "Ethical dilemmas in neurodegenerative disease: Respecting patients at the twilight of agency". In *In Neuroethics: Defining the issues in theory, practice, and policy*. OUP.

Johnston, A. (1997a). "Jacques Lacan". In *Stanford encyclopedia of philosophy*. Stanford University. https://plato.stanford.edu/entries/lacan/#RegThe

Johnston, A. (1997b). "Jaques Lacan". In *Stanford encyclopedia of philosophy*. Stanford University. https://plato.stanford.edu/entries/lacan/#RegThe

Jonze, S. (Director). (1999). *Being John Malkovich*. https://www.imdb.com/title/tt0120601/

Kant, I. (1780). *The Metaphysical Elements of Ethics* (T. K. Abbott, Trans.; Fifth edit). Longmans, Green and Co.

Kant, I., Schneewind, J. B., Baron, M., & Kagan, S. (2002). "Groundwork for the metaphysics of morals with essays". In A. W. Wood (Ed.), *Rethinking the western tradition*. https://doi.org/10.1080/00131857.2014.991501

Karel, M. J., Moye, J., Bank, A., & Azar, A. R. (2007). "Three methods of assessing values for advance care planning: Comparing persons with and without dementia". *Journal of Aging and Health*, 19(1), 123–151. https://doi.org/10.1177/0898264306296394

Karlawish, J. H. T., Casarett, D. J., James, B. D., Xie, S. X., & Kim, S. Y. H. (2005). "The ability of persons with Alzheimer disease (AD) to make a decision about taking an AD treatment". *Neurology*, 64(9), 1514–1519.

Karner, T. X., & Bobbitt-Zeher, D. (2005). "Losing Selves: Dementia Care as Disruption and Transformation". *Symbolic Interaction*, 28(4), 549–570. https://doi.org/10.1525/si.2005.28.4.549

Karnieli-Miller, O., Werner, P., Aharon-Peretz, J., & Eidelman, S. (2007). "Dilemmas in the (un)veiling of the diagnosis of Alzheimer's disease: Walking an ethical and professional tight rope". *Patient Education and Counseling*, 67(3), 307–314.

Katz, S., & Marshall, B. (2003). "New sex for old: Lifestyle, consumerism, and the ethics of aging well". *Journal Of Aging Studies*, 17, 3–16.

Keat, Russell., Whiteley, Nigel., & Abercrombie, Nicholas. (1994). *The Authority of the consumer*. Routledge. https://books.google.com.au/books?hl=en&lr=&id=dtMUqZzOLS0C&oi=fnd&pg=PA53&dq=identity+and+belonging+bauman&ots=I6Sz-Th65rK&sig=VXFl_dtktQVnoQXuDLxKi0732vg#v=onepage&q=identity and belonging bauman&f=false

Kim, D. H. (1999). *Introduction to Systems Thinking*. Pegasus Communications. http://www.thinking.net/Systems_Thinking/Intro_to_ST/intro_to_st.html

Kim, S. Y. H. (2010). *Evaluation of capacity to consent to treatment and research*. Oxford University Press.

Kimbell, B., Boyd, K., Kendall, M., Iredale, J., & Murray, S. (2015). "Managing uncertainty in advanced liver disease: A qualitative, multiperspective serial interview study". *BMJ Open*, 5. http://bmjopen.bmj.com/content/bmjopen/5/11/e009241.full.pdf

Kimbell, B., Murray, S. A., Macpherson, S., & Boyd, K. (2016). "Embracing inherent uncertainty in advanced illness Challenge for people with advanced conditions". *BMJ (Clinical Research Ed.)*, 354(613). https://doi.org/10.1136/bmj.i3802

Kinsella, E. A. (2006). "Hermeneutics and critical hermeneutics: Exploring possibilities within the art of interpretation". *Qualitative Social Research*, 7(3).

Kitwood, T. (1997). "The experience of dementia". *Aging & Mental Health*, 1(1), 13–22. https://doi.org/10.1080/13607869757344

Kitwood, T. (2019). *Dementia Reconsidered Revisited: The person still comes first* (D. Brooker, Ed.; Second edi). OUP Oxford.

Kitwood, T., & Bredin, K. (1992). "Towards a Theory of Dementia Care: Personhood and Well-being". *Ageing and Society*, *12*(3), 269–287.

Komesaroff, P. A. (2008a). *Experiments in Love and Death: Medicine, Postmodernism, Microethics and the Body*. Melbourne University Press.

Komesaroff, P. A. (2008b). "Fardels of the heart". In *Experiments in Love and Death: Medicine, Postmodernism, Microethics and the Body* (pp. 226–246). Melbourne University Press.

Kontos, P. C. (2005). "Embodied selfhood in Alzheimer's disease: Re-thinking person-centred care". *Dementia*, *4*(4), 553–570. https://doi.org/10.1177/1471301205058311

Kontos, P. C. (2006). "Embodied selfhood: An ethnographic exploration of Alzheimer's disease". In A. Leibing & L. Cohen (Eds.), *Thinking about dementia: Culture, loss and the anthropology of senility*. Rutgers University Press.

Kristeva, J. (1982). *Powers of Horror: An Essay on Abjection* (L. S. Roudiez, Trans.). Columbia University Press.

Kurz, A. F., & Lautenschlager, N. T. (2009). "The concept of dementia: Retain, reframe, rename or replace?" *International Psychogeriatrics*, *22*(01), 37. https://doi.org/10.1017/S1041610209991013

Lai, R. (2019). *Pie in the sky*. Walker Books.

Lane, H. P., McLachlan, S., & Philip, J. (2013). "The war against dementia: Are we battle weary yet?" *Age and Ageing*, *42*(3), 281–283. https://doi.org/10.1093/ageing/aft011

Langridge, R., & Christian-Smith, J. (2006). "Access and resilience: Analysing the construction of social resilience to the threat of water scarcity". *Ecology And Society*, *11*(2). http://www.ecologyandsociety.org/vol11/iss2/art18/main.html

Lee, D. (2000). "The Society of Society: The Grand Finale of Niklas Luhmann". *Sociological Theory*, *18*(July), 320–330. https://doi.org/10.1111/0735-2751.00102

Lee, M. J. H. (2010). "The problem of 'thick in status, thin in content' in Beauchamp and Childress' principlism". *Journal of Medical Ethics*, *36*(9), 525–528. https://doi.org/10.1136/jme.2009.031054

Lemmens, C. (2012). "End-of-Life Decisions and Demented Patients. What to Do if the Patient's Current and Past Wishes Are in Conflict with Each Other?" *European Journal of Health Law*, *19*(2), 177–186. https://doi.org/10.1163/157180912x629117

Levinas, E. (1981). *Otherwise Than Being Or Beyond Essence*. Nijhoff. http://books.google.com.au/books?id=18tg1ZHkmTsC

Lieberman, M. A, & Fisher, L. (1999). "The effects of family conflict resolution and decision making on the provision of help for an elder with Alzheimer's disease". *The Gerontologist*, *39*(2), 159–166. https://doi.org/10.1093/geront/39.2.159

Lindemann, H. (2014). *Holding and Letting Go: The Social Practice of Personal Identities*. OUP. https://books.google.com.au/books/about/Holding_and_Letting_Go.html?id=qXT1AQAAQBAJ&redir_esc=y

Lingis, A. (1994). *The Community of Those who Have Nothing in Common*. Indiana University Press. https://books.google.com/books?id=arI1kHTxQTMC&pgis=1

Locke, J. (1764). *The second treatise of Civil Government*. eBooks@Adelaide.

Locke, J. (2015). *An Essay Concerning Human Understanding*. eBooks@Adelaide. https://ebooks.adelaide.edu.au/l/locke/john/l81u/complete.html

Loewy, E. H. (2005). "In Defense of Paternalism". *Theoretical Medicine and Bioethics*, *26*(6), 445–468. https://doi.org/10.1007/s11017-005-2203-0

Logie, R. H., Cocchini, G., Delia Sala, S., & Baddeley, A. D. (2004). "Is there a specific executive capacity for dual task coordination? Evidence from Alzheimer's disease". *Neuropsychology*, *18*(3), 504.

Lopez, R. P., Amella, E. J., Mitchell, S. L., & Strumpf, N. E. (2010). "Nurses' perspectives on feeding decisions for nursing home residents with advanced dementia". *Journal of Clinical Nursing*, *19*(5–6), 632–638. https://doi.org/10.1111/j.1365-2702.2009.03108.x

Luhmann, N. (1992). "What is Communication?" *Forum*, *2*(3), 251–259. https://doi.org/10.1111/j.1468-2885.1992.tb00042.x

Luhmann, N. (2014a). "Contradiction and Conflict". In *Social Systems* (pp. 1–13). Stanford University Press.

Luhmann, N. (2014b). "System and Function". In *Social Systems* (pp. 1–14). Stanford University Press.

Lyotard, J. F. (1979). "The postmodern condition: A report on knowledge". In *The Postmodern Turn*. University of Minnesota Press.

MacIntyre, A. (1981). *After Virtue: A Study in Moral Theory*. Duckworth. http://books.google.com.au/books?id=CoUlAQAAIAAJ

Mackenzie, Catriona., & Stoljar, N. (2000). *Relational autonomy: Feminist perspectives on autonomy, agency, and the social self*. Oxford University Press.

Maturana, H. R. (1974). "The Organisation of the Living: A Theory of the Living Organisation". *Int. J. Human-Computer Studies*, *51*(June 1974), 149–168. https://doi.org/10.1016/S0020-7373(75)80015-0

Maturana, H., & Varela, F. (1980). *Autopoiesis and cognition: The realisation of living*. D. Reidel Publishing Company.

McCormick, R. A. (1999). "Bioethics: A moral vacuum?" *America*, *180*(15), 8–12.

McKenna, M., & Coates, D. J. (2015). *Compatibilism*. Stanford Encyclopedia of Philosophy. https://plato.stanford.edu/entries/compatibilism/

McKhann, G. M., Knopman, D. S., Chertkow, H., Hyman, B. T., Jack, C. R., Kawas, C. H., Klunk, W. E., Koroshetz, W. J., Manly, J. J., Mayeux, R., Mohs, R. C., Morris, J. C., Rossor, M. N., Scheltens, P., Carrillo, M. C., Thies, B., Weintraub, S., & Phelps, C. H. (2011). "The diagnosis of dementia due to Alzheimer's disease: Recommendations from the National Institute on Aging-Alzheimer's Association workgroups on diagnostic guidelines for Alzheimer's disease". *Alzheimer's and Dementia*, *7*(3), 263–269. https://doi.org/10.1016/j.jalz.2011.03.005

McMahan, R. D., Tellez, I., & Sudore, R. (2021). "Deconstructing the Complexities of Advance Care Planning Outcomes: What Do We Know and Where Do We Go? A Scoping Review". *JAGS*, *69*. https://doi.org/DOI: 10.1111/jgs.16801

Meadows, Donella. (2008). *Thinking in systems: A primer*. Chelsea Green Publishing. https://books.google.com.au/books/about/Thinking_in_Systems.html?id=JS-gOSP1qklUC&redir_esc=y

Meilaender, G. (1995). *Body, Soul, and Bioethics*. University of Notre Dame Press. https://books.google.com.au/books/about/Body_Soul_and_Bioethics.html?id=h34rAAAAYAAJ&pgis=1

Menne, H. L., Kinney, J. M., & Morhardt, D. J. (2002). "'Trying to Continue to Do as Much as They Can Do': Theoretical insights regarding continuity and meaning making in the face of dementia". *Dementia*, *1*(3), 367–382. https://doi.org/10.1177/147130120200100308

Menne, H. L., Tucke, S. S., Whitlatch, C. J., & Feinberg, L. F. (2008). "Decision-making involvement scale for individuals with dementia and family caregivers". *American Journal of Alzheimer's Disease and Other Dementias*, *23*(1), 23–29. https://doi.org/10.1177/1533317507308312

Merleau-Ponty, M., & Smith, C. (2005). *Phenomenology of Perception*. Taylor and Francis eLibrary.

Mill, J. S. (1859). *On Liberty*. Batoche Books. https://socialsciences.mcmaster.ca/econ/ugcm/3ll3/mill/liberty.pdf

Mitchell, D. T., & Snyder, S. (2016). "The Matter of Disability". *Journal of Bioethical Inquiry*. https://doi.org/10.1007/s11673-016-9740-2

Modi, S. C., Whetstone, L. M., & Cummings, D. M. (2007). "Influence of patient and physician characteristics on percutaneous endoscopic gastrostomy tube decision-making". *Journal Of Palliative Medicine*, *10*(2), 359–366.

Moeller, H. (2005). *Luhmann explained: From souls to systems*. http://books.google.com.au/books?hl=en&lr=&id=tuKsEvpcj9MC&oi=fnd&pg=PR9&ots=TmQvp-1x2t&sig=-5JGVgqYXW-4zyD1-CrbdHK85SuU

Moody, H. R. (1996). *Ethics in an Aging Society*. Johns Hopkins University Press. http://www.amazon.com/Ethics-Aging-Society-Harry-Moody/dp/0801853974

Morgan, T., Ann Williams, L., Trussardi, G., & Gott, M. (2016). "Gender and family caregiving at the end-of-life in the context of old age: A systematic review". *Palliative Medicine*. https://doi.org/10.1177/0269216315625857

Morris, S. (2018). "'THE TORMENT OF OUR POWERLESSNESS': ADDRESSING INDIGENOUS CONSTITUTIONAL VULNERABILITY THROUGH THE ULURU STATEMENT'S CALL FOR A FIRST NATIONS VOICE IN THEIR AFFAIRS". *UNSW Law Journal*, *41*(3). https://www.unswlawjournal.unsw.edu.au/wp-content/uploads/2018/09/Morris.pdf

Morton, I. (2001). *Person-centred approaches to dementia care*. Speechmark.

Muramoto, O. (2011). "Socially and temporally extended end-of-life decision-making process for dementia patients". *Journal of Medical Ethics*, *37*(6), 339–343. https://doi.org/10.1136/jme.2010.038950

Murray, S. a, Kendall, M., Boyd, K., & Sheikh, A. (2005). "Illness trajectories and palliative care". *BMJ (Clinical Research Ed.)*, *330*, 1007–1011. https://doi.org/10.1136/bmj.330.7498.1007

Nedelsky, J. (2011). *Law's Relations: A Relational Theory of Self, Autonomy, and Law*. Oxford University Press, USA. https://books.google.com/books?hl=en&lr=&id=TbfD-8mtW-LIC&pgis=1

Nolan, M., Brown, J., Davies, S., Nolan, J., & Keady, J. (2006). *The Senses Framework: Improving care for older people through a relationship-centred approach. Getting Research into Practice (GRiP) Report No 2. Project* (2). Sheffield Hallam University.

Nolan, M., Davies, S., & Brown, J. (2006). "Transitions in care homes: Towards relationship-centred care using the 'Senses Framework'". *Quality in Ageing*, *7*(3), 5–15. https://doi.org/10.1108/14717794200600015

Nolan, M., Ryan, T., Enderby, P., & Reid, D. (2002). "Towards a More Inclusive Vision of Dementia Care Practice and Research". *Dementia, 1*(2), 193–211. https://doi.org/10.1177/147130120200100206

Nussbaum, M. C. (2004). *Hiding from Humanity: Disgust, Shame, and the Law*. Princeton University Press. https://books.google.com/books?id=XfSYON-JXHwC&pgis=1

Nussbaum, M. C. (2009). *Frontiers of justice: Disability, nationality, species membership.*

Okonkwo, O. C., Griffith, H. R., Belue, K., Lanza, S., Zamrini, E. Y., Harrell, L. E., Brockington, J. C., Clark, D., Raman, R., & Marson, D. C. (2008). "Cognitive models of medical decision-making capacity in patients with mild cognitive impairment". *Journal Of The International Neuropsychological Society: JINS, 14*(2), 297–308. https://doi.org/10.1017/s1355617708080338

Okonkwo, O. C., Griffith, H. R., Copeland, J. N., Belue, K., Lanza, S., Zamrini, E. Y., Harrell, L. E., Brockington, J. C., Clark, D., Raman, R., & Marson, D. C. (2008). "Medical decision-making capacity in mild cognitive impairment: A 3-year longitudinal study". *Neurology, 71*(19), 1474–1480. https://doi.org/10.1212/01.wnl.0000334301.32358.48

Okonkwo, O., Griffith, H. R., Belue, K., Lanza, S., Zamrini, E. Y., Harrell, L. E., Brockington, J. C., Clark, D., Raman, R., & Marson, D. C. (2007). "Medical decision-making capacity in patients with mild cognitive impairment". *Neurology, 69*(15), 1528–1535.

Oliveira, C. C. (2013). "What Bateson had in Mind About 'Mind'"? *Biosemiotics, 6*(3), 515–536. https://doi.org/10.1007/s12304-013-9190-8

O'Neill, N., & Peisah, C. (2011)." Chapter 1 – Capacity". In *Capacity and the law* (pp. 1–10). AustLII communities. http://austlii.community/wiki/Books/CapacityAndTheLaw/

Oshana, M. (2006). *Personal Autonomy in Society*. Ashgate Publishing, Ltd. https://books.google.com.au/books/about/Personal_Autonomy_in_Society.html?id=K-CRAKsgGME4C&pgis=1

Oshana, M. A. L. (1998). "Personal autonomy and society". *Journal of Social Philosophy, 29*(1), 81–102. https://doi.org/10.1111/j.1467-9833.1998.tb00098.x

Packer, T. (2000). Does person-centred care exist. *Journal of Dementia Care, 8*(3). http://www.scie-socialcareonline.org.uk/does-person-centred-care-exist/r/a1CG-0000000GQx0MAG

Panza, F., Lozupone, M., Logroscino, G., & Imbimbo, B. P. (2019). "A critical appraisal of amyloid-targeting therapies for Alzheimer disease". *Nature Reviews Neurology, 15*(2), 73–88. https://doi.org/10.1038/s41582-018-0116-6

Parfit, D. (1984). *Reasons and Persons*. OUP Oxford. https://books.google.com.au/books/about/Reasons_and_Persons.html?id=i5wQaJI3668C&pgis=1

Parker, D. (2011). "Residential Aged Care Facilities Places for Living and Dying". *Cultural Studies Review, 17*(1), 31–51.

Parmenidou, A. V. (2011). "Second-Order Change in Psychotherapy: A Necessary Requirement? Remaining sane in insane places". *16th International Conference of A.P.P.A.C.*, 1–14.

Pasman, H. R. W., Mei, B. A., Onwuteaka-Philipsen, B. D., Ribbe, M. W., & van der Wal, G. (2004). "Participants in the decision-making on artificial nutrition and hydration to demented nursing home patients: A qualitative study". *Journal Of Aging Studies, 18*(3), 321–335. https://doi.org/10.1016/j.jaging.2004.03.003

Patrick, D. L., Starks, H. E., Cain, K. C., Uhlmann, R. F., & Pearlman, R. A. (1994). "Measuring preferences for health states worse than death". *Medical Decision Making: An International Journal Of The Society For Medical Decision Making*, *14*(1), 9–18.

Peisah, C., Sorinmade, O. a, Mitchell, L., & Hertogh, C. M. P. M. (2013). "Decisional capacity: Toward an inclusionary approach". *International Psychogeriatrics / IPA*, *25*(10), 1571–1579. https://doi.org/10.1017/S1041610213001014

Phillipson, L., Magee, C., Jones, S., & Skladzien, E. (2012). *Exploring dementia and stigma beliefs: A pilot study of adults aged 40 to 65 years* (Issue 28). Alzheimer's Australia.

Phinney, A., Kelson, E., Baumbusch, J., OConnor, D., & Purves, B. (2016). "Walking in the neighbourhood: Performing social citizenship in dementia". *Dementia*, *15*(3), 381–394. https://doi.org/10.1177/1471301216638180

Pierce, C. (2000). *Hard to Forget: An Alzheimer's Story*. Random House Publishing Group. http://books.google.com.au/books?id=Q1osAAAAYAAJ

Plassman, B. L., Williams, J. W., Burke, J. R., Holsinger, T., & Benjamin, S. (2010). "Systematic review: Factors associated with risk for and possible prevention of cognitive decline in later life". *Annals of Internal Medicine*, *153*(3), 182–193. https://doi.org/10.7326/0003-4819-153-3-201008030-00258

Popper, K. R. (1962). *Conjectures and Refutations: The Growth of Scientific Knowledge* (Vol. 2nd). Basic Books.

Post, S. G. (2006). "Respectare: Moral respect for the lives of the deeply forgetful". In J. C. Hughes, S. J. Louw, & S. R. Sabat (Eds.), *Dementia: Mind, meaning and person* (pp. 223–235). Oxford University Press. http://oxfordmedicine.com/view/10.1093/med/9780198566151.001.0001/med-9780198566151-chapter-014

Proust, M. (1982). *Remembrance of Things Past Volume 1*. Vintage. https://www.amazon.com/Remembrance-Things-Past-Volumes-1-3/dp/0394712439

Quill, T. E., & Brody, H. (1996). "Physician recommendations and patient autonomy: Finding a balance between physician power and patient choice". *Annals of Internal Medicine*, *125*(9), 763–769.

Rawls, J. (1999). *Collected Papers—John Rawls, Samuel Freeman* (S. Freeman, Ed.). Harvard University Press. https://www.hup.harvard.edu/catalog.php?isbn=9780674137394

Rawls, J. (2005). *Political liberalism*. Columbia University Press.

Rawls, J. (2006). "A Theory of Justice: Revised Edition". In *Cambridge, MA: Belknap* (Vol. 5). http://www.mediafire.com/?cj2zlxccc3fuc14%5Cnpapers2://publication/uuid/B4578407-EBD9-4370-A473-357C20C3DF33

Ribolsi, M., Feyaerts, J., & Vanhuele, S. (2015.). "Metaphor in psychosis: On the possible convergence of Lacanian theory and neuro-scientific research". *Frontiers in Psychiatry*, *6*. https://doi.org/10.3389/fpsyg.2015.00664

Richards, M., & Brayne, C. (2010). "What do we mean by Alzheimer's disease? Challenges to the pathology-led view". *BMJ: British Medical Journal*, *4670*(October), 1–5. https://doi.org/10.1136/bmj.c4670

Richter, J., Eisemann, M., & Zgonnikova, E. (2001). "Doctors' authoritarianism in end-of-life treatment decisions. A comparison between Russia, Sweden and Germany". *Journal Of Medical Ethics*, *27*(3), 186–191.

Ricoeur, P. (1995). *Oneself as Another* (K. Blamey, Trans.). University of Chicago Press.

Ricoeur, P., & Escobar, M. (2004). "Otherwise: A Reading of Emmanuel Levinas's 'Otherwise than Being or beyond Essence'". *Yale French Studies*, *104*, 82–99. https://doi.org/10.2307/3182506

Ries, N. M., Thompson, K. A., & Lowe, M. (2017). "Including People with Dementia in Research: An Analysis of Australian Ethical and Legal Rules and Recommendations for Reform". *Journal of Bioethical Inquiry*, *14*(3), 359–374. https://doi.org/10.1007/s11673-017-9794-9

Rogers, C. R. (Carl R.) (1995). *On becoming a person: A therapist's view of psychotherapy*. Houghton Mifflin.

Rosow, K., Holzapfel, A., Karlawish, J. H., Baumgart, M., Bain, L. J., & Khachaturian, A. S. (2011). "Countrywide strategic plans on Alzheimer's disease: Developing the framework for the international battle against Alzheimer's disease". *Alzheimer's & Dementia*, *7*(6), 615–621. https://doi.org/10.1016/j.jalz.2011.09.226

Rubinstein, R. L., & De Medeiros, K. (2015). "'Successful Aging,' Gerontological theory and neoliberalism: A qualitative critique". *Gerontologist*, *55*(1), 34–42. https://doi.org/10.1093/geront/gnu080

Rurup, M. L., Onwuteaka-Philipsen, B. D., Pasman, H. R. W., Ribbe, M. W., & van der Wal, G. (2006). "Attitudes of physicians, nurses and relatives towards end-of-life decisions concerning nursing home patients with dementia". *Patient Education and Counseling*, *61*(3), 372–380. https://doi.org/10.1016/j.pec.2005.04.016

Sabat, S. R. (2002). "Surviving Manifestations of Selfhood in Alzheimer's Disease: A case study". *Dementia*, *1*(1), 25–36. https://doi.org/10.1177/147130120200100101

Sabat, S. R., & Harré, R. (1992). "The Construction and Deconstruction of Self in Alzheimer's Disease". *Ageing and Society*, *12*(04), 443. https://doi.org/10.1017/S0144686X00005262

Sachdev, P. S., Blacker, D., Blazer, D. G., Ganguli, M., Jeste, D. V., Paulsen, J. S., & Petersen, R. C. (2014). "Classifying neurocognitive disorders: The DSM-5 approach". *Nature Reviews Neurology*, *10*(11), Article 11. https://doi.org/10.1038/nrneurol.2014.181

Scheidt, R. J., Bosch, J. V., Kivnick, H. Q., & Bosch, J. V. (2015). "Filming 'Successful Aging'". *The Gerontologist*, 55(1), 169–170. https://doi.org/10.1093/geront/gnu172

Schneider, J. A., Arvanitakis, Z., Leurgans, S. E., & Bennett, D. A. (2009). "The neuropathology of probable Alzheimer disease and mild cognitive impairment". *Annals of Neurology*, *66*(2), 200–208. https://doi.org/10.1002/ana.21706

Sherwin, S. (Ed.). (1998). *The Politics of Women's Health: Exploring Agency and Autonomy*. Temple University Press.

Shoemaker, D. (2015). "Personal Identity". In *Stanford Encyclopedia of Philosophy*. https://plato.stanford.edu/entries/identity-personal/

Simmel, G. (1950). *The sociology of Georg Simmel*. Simon and Schuster.

Slaughter, S., Cole, D., Jennings, E., & Reimer, M. (2007). "Consent and Assent to Participate in Research from People with Dementia". *Nursing Ethics*, *14*(1).

Smith, A. (2009). "Decision-Making as Social Practice: Exploring the relevance of Bourdieu's Concepts of Habitus and Symbolic Capital". In D. O'Connor & B. A. Purves (Eds.), *Decision-Making, Personhood and Dementia: Exploring the Interface* (pp. 37–46). Jessica Kingsley Publishers.

Soo Parl, Y., Konge, L., & Artino, A. R. (2020). "The Positivism Paradigm of Research". *Academic Medicine*, *95*(5).

Spalding, N. J., & Phillips, T. (2007). "Exploring the Use of Vignettes: From Validity to Trustworthiness". *Qualitative Health Research, 17*(7), 954–962. https://doi.org/10.1177/1049732307306187

Spike, J. P. (2007). "Responding to requests for dialysis for severely demented and brain injured patients". *Seminars in Dialysis, 20*(5), 387–390.

Steeman, E., Godderis, J., Grypdonck, M., De Bal, N., & De Casterlé, B. D. (2007). "Living with dementia from the perspective of older people: Is it a positive story?" *Aging & Mental Health, 11*(2), 119–130. https://doi.org/10.1080/13607860600963364

Stern, D. N. (1998). *The Interpersonal World of the Infant: A View from Psychoanalysis and Developmental Psychology*. Karnac Books. https://books.google.com/books?id=4yHiUkgKlvUC&pgis=1

Stewart, R. (2006). "Mental health legislation and decision making capacity: Autonomy in Alzheimer's disease is ignored and neglected". *BMJ (Clinical Research Ed.), 332*(7533), 118–119. https://doi.org/10.1136/bmj.332.7533.118-b

Stoljar, N. (2013). "Feminist Perspectives on Autonomy". In *Stanford Encyclopedia of Philosophy*. https://plato.stanford.edu/entries/feminism-autonomy/#RelAut

Sugarman, J., Cain, C., Wallace, R., & Welsh-Bohmer, K. A. (2001). "How proxies make decisions about research for patients with Alzheimer's disease". *Journal Of The American Geriatrics Society, 49*(8), 1110–1119. https://doi.org/10.1046/j.1532-5415.2001.49218.x

Summa, M., & Fuchs, T. (2015). "Self-experience in Dementia". *Rivista Internazionale Di Filosofia e Psicologia, 6*(2), 387–405. https://doi.org/10.4453/rifp.2015.0038

Szejnwald Brown, H., & Vergragt, P. J. (2016). "From consumerism to wellbeing: Toward a cultural transition?" *Journal of Cleaner Production, 132*, 308–317. http://dx.doi.org/10.1016/j.jclepro.2015.04.107

Taylor, C. (1989). *Sources of the self: The making of modern identity*. Harvard University Press.

Taylor, C. (2012). "Foucault and familial power". *Hypatia, 27*(1). https://www.jstor.org/stable/41328905

Taylor, J. S. (2005a). "Introduction". In J. S. Taylor (Ed.), *Personal Autonomy: New essays on personal autonomy and its role in contemporary moral philosophy*. Cambridge University Press. https://doi.org/10.1111/1467-9973.00225

Taylor, J. S. (Ed.). (2005b). *Personal autonomy: New essays on personal autonomy and its role in contemporary moral philosophy*. Cambridge University Press.

Torralva, T., Dorrego, F., Sabe, L., Chemerinski, E., & Starkstein, S. E. (2000). "Impairments of social cognition and decision making in Alzheimer's disease". *International Psychogeriatrics, 12*(3), 359–368. https://doi.org/10.1017/S1041610200006463

Tronto, J. (2020). *Moral Boundaries: A Political Argument for an Ethic of Care*. Routledge. https://doi.org/10.4324/9781003070672

Turteltaub, J. (Director). (2016). *Las Vegas*. Good Universe.

Tyrrell, J., Genin, N., & Myslinski, M. (2006). "Freedom of choice and decision-making in health and social care". *Dementia: The International Journal of Social Research and Practice, 5*(4), 479–502. https://doi.org/10.1177/1471301206069915

van der Steen, J. T., Helton, M. R., & Ribbe, M. W. (2009). "Prognosis is important in decision-making in Dutch nursing home patients with dementia and pneumonia". *International Journal of Geriatric Psychiatry, 24*(9), 933–936. https://doi.org/10.1002/gps.2198

van der Steen, J. T., van der Wal, G., Mehr, D. R., Ooms, M. E., & Ribbe, M. W. (2005). "End-of-Life Decision Making in Nursing Home Residents with Dementia and Pneumonia: Dutch Physicians' Intentions Regarding Hastening Death". *Alzheimer Disease and Associated Disorders*, *19*(3), 148–155. https://doi.org/10.1097/01.wad.0000175525.99104.b7

van der Steen, J. T., & Volicer, L. (2011). "Decision-making in patients with severe dementia and pneumonia: Cross-national perspectives". *International Journal Of Geriatric Psychiatry*, *26*(2), 216–217. https://doi.org/10.1002/gps.2542

Walters, J. W. (1997). *What is a person?: An ethical exploration*. University of Illinois Press.

Wang, R.-S. (2013). "Perturbation". In *Encyclopedia of Systems Biology* (pp. 1680–1681). Springer New York. https://doi.org/10.1007/978-1-4419-9863-7_385

Watson, J. (2019.). "Developing the Senses Framework to support relationship-centred care for people with advanced dementia until the end of life in care homes". *Dementia*, *18*(2), 545–566. https://doi.org/10.1177/1471301216682880

Whitehouse, P. J. (1985). "Theodor Meynert: Foreshadowing modern concepts of neuropsychiatric pathophysiology". *Neurology*, *35*(3), 389–391.

Whitlatch, C. J., & Menne, H. L. (2009). "Don't forget about me! Decision making by people with dementia". *Generations*, *33*(1), 66–73.

Williams, L. A., Giddings, L. S., Bellamy, G., & Gott, M. (2017). "'Because it's the wife who has to look after the man': A descriptive qualitative study of older women and the intersection of gender and the provision of family caregiving at the end of life". *Palliative Medicine*, *31*(3), 223–230. https://doi.org/10.1177/0269216316653275

Wolf, S. (1993). *Freedom within Reason*. Oxford University Press.

Xu, L., Marinova, D., & Guo, X. (2015). "Resilience thinking: A renewed system approach for sustainability science". *Sustainability Science*, *10*(1), 123–138. https://doi.org/10.1007/s11625-014-0274-4

Young, R. B. (1986). *Personal Autonomy: Beyond negative and positive liberty*. Crrom Helm.

Zahavi, D. (2005). *Subjectivity and Selfhood: Investigating the First-Person Perspective*. MIT Press.

Zeilig, H. (2014). "Dementia As a Cultural Metaphor". *The Gerontologist*, *54*(2), 258–267. https://doi.org/10.1093/geront/gns203

Žižek, Slavoj. (2006a). *How to read Lacan*. Granta.

Žižek, Slavoj. (2006b). *The parallax view*. MIT Press. https://books.google.com.au/books/about/The_Parallax_View.html?id=je702bo2Pl8C

Zournazi, M., & Wenders, Wi. (2013). *Inventing Peace: A Dialogue on Perception*. I.B. Tauris. https://books.google.com.au/books/about/Inventing_Peace.html?id=4Vc-JAwAAQBAJ&redir_esc=y

• • •

Index

S

T

U

V

W

Z

www.ingramcontent.com/pod-product-compliance
Lightning Source LLC
Chambersburg PA
CBHW060029030426

42334CB00019B/2246